Alkaline Diet for Beginners:

The Best Guide to Understand PH; Learn How to Improve Your Weight Loss in A Healthy and Natural Way; Create A New Unlimited Energy Lifestyle To Reset and Cleanse Your Body

By Julie Water

The reproduction, transmission, and duplication of any of the content found herein, including any specific or extended information will be done as an illegal act regardless of the end form the information ultimately takes. This includes copied versions of the work both physical, digital and audio unless express consent of the Publisher is provided beforehand. Any additional rights reserved.

Furthermore, the information that can be found within the pages described forthwith shall be considered both accurate and truthful when it comes to the recounting of facts. As such, any use, correct or incorrect, of the provided information will render the Publisher free of responsibility as to the actions taken outside of their direct purview. Regardless, there are zero scenarios where the original author or the Publisher can be deemed liable in any fashion for any damages or hardships that may result from any of the information discussed herein.

Additionally, the information in the following pages is intended only for informational purposes and should thus be thought of as universal. As befitting its nature, it is presented without assurance regarding its prolonged validity or interim quality. Trademarks that are mentioned are done without written consent and can in no way be considered an endorsement from the trademark holder.

Table of contents

Start Easy

Introduction

Thank you so much for downloading *The Best Guide to Understand PH; Learn How to Improve Your Weight Loss in A Healthy and Natural Way; Create A New Unlimited Energy In Lifestyle To Reset and Cleanse Your Body*. In this book, we're going to be talking about the alkaline diet, and what it can do for you in terms of providing you with better overall health and to help you live a long life. You might have heard of the alkaline diet, and it is, in fact, the most popular diet in today's day and age.

The reason why is because it works, even though many people consider the alkaline diet as a relatively difficulty diet to continue with, it is still one of the most rewarding and fantastic diet's out there. In this book, we are going to be talking about the alkaline diet, and what it can do for you both mentally, physically, and internally. Many diets only cover the physical part. Whereas, the alkaline diet includes all three, making this diet an ideal diet for people who are looking for the life-changing results.

That being said, once you are done with this book you will have a great idea on how to follow the alkaline diet but more specifically, understand how this diet can change your life for the better. If anything seems overwhelming for you in this book, reread it and try to understand it. Trust me, and if you read it once more, then you will have a better idea on what the content is trying to convey.

Are you looking to change the way your body feels once in for all and to start seeing better results? If so we have the answer for you. The alkaline diet is one of the best diets to change the way your body functions and to help you get the best results possible without making you spend too much. Contrary to popular belief, the alkaline diet could be one of the least expensive diets to follow and can help you tremendously in regards to bettering your health and well-being.

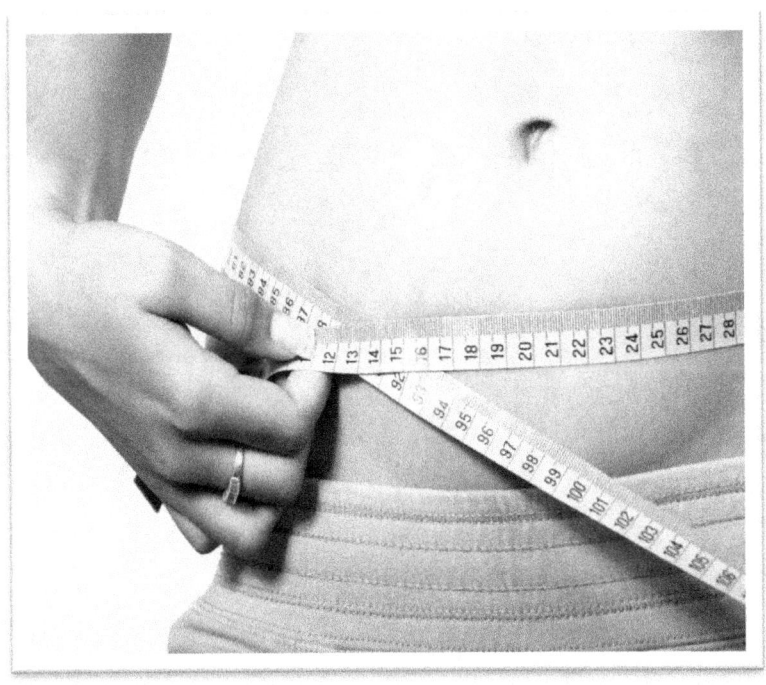

Chapter 1: What Is the Alkaline Diet

Many people who are looking to stay healthy and to see better results overall, will do whatever it takes to achieve optimal health and wellness - which is why, many people follow diets such as intermittent fasting, ketogenic diet, and many more. Even though these diets work great when it comes to losing weight, and to see better results overall. That does not mean, you will not see the benefits which you are looking for. On the other hand, the alkaline diet provides you with amazing results such as better health, better physique, and just better bodily functions overall. Even though you are aware of the benefits which come along the alkaline diet, you still need to understand the basics of the alkaline diet and how it can help you. The first thing we will talk about is what is the alkaline diet, and what it requires you to do.

The alkaline diet is simply a diet, where you will be paying close attention to your pH level to ensure that you are staying at an alkaline state. There are two states in our body acidic and alkaline. The main thing you have to keep in mind when following the diet is for you to say at an alkaline state. Which is why it is essential that you eat foods which will help you stay at an alkaline state, in later chapters were going to talk about the foods that are alkaline and acidic but just keep in mind, that for you to achieve optimal success with this diet your goal should be to say alkaline most of the time. Based on the pH level, your pH level should be at 7.5 pH for you to be at an alkaline state, we will talk about the pH levels later on in this book as well. The reason why the alkaline diet started was to help people live a healthier life and to get rid of tons of diseases that we are facing in the modern day and age.

Most of the problems and diseases are caused by the acidic environment. What diseases love is an acidic environment, which is why the alkaline diet works so great in order to get rid of harmful bacteria and diseases. Even though this diet is primarily based on you getting rid of any diseases that you might be facing; it is still important to understand that your physical appearance will change once you start following this diet. The reason why your appearance will change when you start following this diet is very simple; most of the very alkaline foods are extremely healthy for you regardless. And for you to overeat when following the alkaline diet would be impossible, which is why this diet works so great in terms of helping you lose weight and to see better health benefits overall. Keep in mind that this diet was not primarily made for aesthetic reasons or for you to look a certain way. The physical appearance changes come naturally with the alkaline diet, but it isn't the main idea behind it.

Furthermore, this diet will be very meticulous when it comes to food selection. As we told you previously, we will give you a full food section where you can pick out the foods that you're going to be eating when following the alkaline diet. However, you need to understand the concept that you will have to give up a lot of foods which you are eating right now. Which is why many people don't follow this diet as it can be very hard to follow. That being said, this should not stop you from following the alkaline diet simply because it is difficult. Even though this diet is complicated, many people who follow this diet have said that not only did this diet help them live a better life, but it also helped them to lower risk of many diseases such as cancer, blood pressure and many more. This diet is truly a great diet to follow if your goal is to see life-changing benefits out of it. Not only that, expect to see amazing results in your physical activities. If you're an athlete or someone looking to gain more notoriety in your athletic performance, then this diet could be a great idea for you.

Many athletes who follow the alkaline diet have said that this diet helped them perform a lot better at their peak performance. It also helped them to perform for a longer period of time. Making this diet a great diet to follow if you're an athlete, and it is also a great diet to follow if you're just a regular Joe. This diet so versatile when it comes to benefits, it could work for an athlete and a regular Joe. Which is why you hear more people talking about the alkaline diet, it is simply that good. Time and time again, many people have said that a diet which you can stick with is the best diet you can follow.

However, if people can stick with the alkaline diet, then it will yield them the best results possible. As we told you previously, many people have issues following this diet for a long period of time, simply because it is so hard to follow and the food restrictions that come along with it. We will give you a lifestyle breakdown that will help you to continue on with this diet without any hiccups, keep in mind that it is essential that you follow this diet for a long period of time. The reason why the diet works at a longer period of time is that the body likes homeostasis. Meaning your body will react better once it is comfortable with being at an alkaline state.

The Alkaline diet will work on some people. The best thing for you to do would be to find out for yourself whether this diet is for you or not, many people look for short and easy answers by looking at the reviews online. Let's talk about some of the diet restrictions or preferences when following the Alkaline diet, and how this diet will most likely be a vegan or vegetarian for the most part. As this diet requires you to eat foods which do not include any meat or any dairy products in them, this makes it a vegan diet overall.

Another thing you needs to be taken care of when following the alkaline diet is that it is supposed to be gluten-free, which means that you need to stay away from as much gluten as possible, which means taking out any wheat products from your diet. You also need to make sure that you are taking out most of the products which have dairy in them, although many people say that eggs are not allowed in the alkaline diet you can still have them at a decent amount. Although this diet has many positives to it, it has one major downfall. The major disadvantage of this diet is that it will be costly for you to follow. The alkaline diet requires you to eat just organic vegetables, which is one of the biggest things of this diet is that you need to make sure the food you're going to be getting is organic.

This could really add up the cost of your diet, another thing you need to take care of when following this diet would be the eating plan. You need to make sure that you are taking the right supplementation in order to take care of your body and to keep it at an alkaline state. Just to clarify, if you don't have the budget for it, then you don't need to buy supplements; however, it is highly recommended that you do so. One of the significant supplements to take in, which will help you with the diet is alkaline water. If you've ever bought alkaline water, then you would know that the alkaline water is costly and can add up in the long run.

This could be considered one of the most essential supplements when following the alkaline diet. However, if you can't afford the diet or the supplement, then we highly recommend you not follow it overall. Sure, there are many ways to cut out the cost in this diet. However, it is still an expensive diet, nonetheless. With that being said, many people will be wondering if this diet is for them or not? Well, let me help you out with that. The right answer would be maybe, now to give you a brief example on how to test out your body's alkaline level is very simple.

There's a pH measuring paper that you can get at any grocery store, basically how you test is you put the strip underneath your tongue, and it will tell you how acidic or alkaline you are, if you're at a zero that means you are totally acidic while if you have 14 that means you're entirely alkaline. Many people tend to fall out between 6 to 8 pH level, 7 being neutral. This is one of the ways to test your alkaline or acidic level, and there are many other ways to test it out like your stomach and your urine sample which changes very frequently, more on that later on in the book. The alkaline diet claims to help your body maintain your blood pH level.

In fact, in this diet, there is nothing that you're going to eat, which will cause imbalances in your pH level and therefore keep your body at a very alkaline level overall. Being alkaline is very important when it comes to lowering the risk of many diseases, for example, if your body is in an acidic environment, then you will attract more of the diseases such as cancer. There have been many cases showing that extremely acidic people, contracted more diseases as compared to people who were on the alkaline side. Being on the alkaline side tends to lower the risk of any diseases, hence making this diet one of the best diets to start following when it comes to keeping good health overall.

Now, besides the meat, you will be cutting out a lot more stuff. You will be cutting out one of the most consumed beverages in the world, and yes, we're talking about caffeinated drinks. If you drink any amount of caffeine, from any source, then it is time for you to cut it out. Unfortunately, caffeine tends to increase the level of acid in your body, therefore, making it unfeasible for people to consume caffeine while following the Alkaline diet. You also need to cut out alcohol from your diet. There have been many studies showing that alcohol also tends to raise acid level in your body, which is why you need to cut out alcohol alongside with your caffeine consumption.

This it could be hard for many people to give up, which is why many people recommend easing into the alkaline diet. Since you will be cutting out a lot of foods which we consume daily, it will make the diet very high effort. You will be eating foods basically for nutrition and helping your body live a healthier life overall. As we said previously, you will be cutting out any comfort foods or any drinks.

Would make you feel better like coffee and alcohol. Be prepared for that when start following this diet, For the people who are confused, let me break it down for you very simply. You will mainly be a vegan when following this diet.

However, you will be more restrictive than a vegan diet. Your diet will be very meticulous when it comes to picking out the right foods, making it impossible for you to eat outside at a restaurant. As we keep saying to you, this diet will be tough to follow in the short term. However, once you start following this diet for a long time, it will become second nature, and you will start living the life you have been dreaming about. Not only that, the great news about this diet is that it will help you lower your blood pressure cholesterol, which is a significant risk factor when it comes to any heart diseases.

As you know, many people face harsh diseases in North American society, which makes this diet one of the best diets to follow when it comes to living a healthier life, especially for North American. This diet will also help you to lower the risk of diabetes and osteoporosis. But one of the best things about this diet is that it will help you recover from cancer. Although not proven, there have been many studies showing that chemotherapy drugs are more effective when having a more alkaline body. And when you have an alkaline body, there's a lower chance of cancer surviving in that body and therefore making it very easy for you to recover from cancer.

If you have any diseases that you need to take care of or need to get rid of, then make sure that you consult with your doctor before you follow any of these diets. Although this diet might help you tremendously and has helped many people, it doesn't mean that it will help you 100 %. Make sure that you talk to your doctor and follow their information, as this book doesn't know how your body functions. We are talking about the mass after you have managed to understand the diet and what it requires, know that this diet can be one of the best things you follow if your goal is to live a healthier life overall. Just remember, that even though this information is very proven and has been backed up, it does not mean that it will work for you.

In fact, just a diet might not be the right answer for you if your goal is simply to lose weight. If your goal is to lose weight, live a healthier life, and live a longer life, then we highly recommend that you follow this diet to make it happen for you. This diet is ideal for people who are looking to change their life internally and externally. If your goal is to follow this diet for aesthetic reasons, then it is recommended that you follow other diets.

There are many diets which would be much easier for you to follow and you will lose a lot of weight. This diet is for people who are already following a healthy diet but are looking to be healthy internally.

Being the diet is advanced, we recommend that you have a specific idea on how to follow diets before you jump into the Alkaline diet as it can be tough for most people to follow. Also, we recommend that you consult with your doctor before you follow any of these diets as some foods in here might not be the right idea for you. This diet is basically for people who are healthy looking to stay healthy for a more extended period of time, and for people who are facing certain diseases and are looking to change.

The environment in their body which will allow them to stay healthy for a more extended period, and also get rid of all the diseases they might be facing.

Chapter 2: Benefits of the Alkaline Diet

The Alkaline diet has a lot of health benefits. Some benefits will surprise you. Nonetheless you will understand and see the reason why many people like following this diet. Make sure you read them, allowing you to understand how this diet can help you in the long run.

Weight-Loss in a Healthy Manner

As you know, there are many ways to lose weight. However, one of the most popular methods being used to lose weight is the Alkaline diet, and there is a good reason behind it. Many people don't know this, but Alkaline diet is perhaps the best way for someone to lose "body fat" instead of "body-weight." When following most diets, followers tend to lose a ton of weight, but most of the time it is muscle and water weight they are getting rid of.

On the other hand, the Alkaline diet makes you lose more body fat. Here is how it works, when you are eating right healthy foods for a prolonged period you have burned out all your glycogen stores, as your caloric intake drops. Which makes the body hit your reserves, and that of course, is your body fat. You will be burning more body fat, instead of muscle mass or glycogen, which makes it ideal for people looking to lose weight. Also, as you know, proper diet plays a huge role in affecting your hormones. Your insulin will flatline, and your growth hormone will go up, this will prime your body to burn body fat instead and will do so in a healthy manner.

Increased Longevity

There have been many studies showing that the Alkaline diet can boost endurance. As you might know by now that alkaline diet can help you with cell rejuvenation or also known as autophagy, this process enables you to get rid of the old and weak cell and replace it with newer stronger ones. This process has shown to increase longevity and overall well-being, which is one of the reasons why the Alkaline diet can help you live a longer life. Moreover, some studies are showing that reducing calories in animals by 30% to 40% has shown to increase their lifespan. However, there is no study done on humans claiming such.

Nonetheless, some studies are suggesting that monkeys that ate less food but more on the alkaline side lived longer. However, there was another study indicating that it wasn't the case on 25-year-old long research done by another party.

Although there is no actual study backing these claims up, it does show that people who ate less had a fewer risk of diseases which could lead to longevity. Which is excellent news when looking at it from that angle, there is a lot of disease prevention that comes with the Alkaline diet, but we will talk about those later in this chapter. However, the main thing to remember would be the fact that Alkaline diet helps with autophagy, which enables you to rejuvenate cells, which makes it very evident that the Alkaline diet can help you with longevity and overall well-being, which is a great thing to consider.

Prevent Diseases

There are many diseases present in today's day and age, and it very common to meet someone suffering from one. Which means, we need to figure out a way to reduce the risk of diseases for overall health and well-being. The alkaline diet has shown to lower risk of many diseases, and we will be discussing all the disorders the Alkaline diet can help get rid of. One of the many conditions Alkaline diet could help manage would be Alzheimer's and Parkinson's.

As you know, the Alkaline diet helps with boost brain health and to lower the risk of neurologic diseases. Some studies are showing that the Alkaline diet can help reduce the risk of depression, even though some people might not consider this a condition, it is still a significant issue in our society. The alkaline diet has also shown to reduce cholesterol, a 2010 study on overweight women found that the alkaline diet improved hosts of health complications including cholesterol levels (LDL) and blood pressure which is also known as the silent killer.

The Alkaline diet also helps with reducing type 2 diabetes, and there was one study done on men, which showed that Alkaline helped them stop insulin treatment. Although we don't recommend, you try this if you have type 2 diabetes, that goes to show you the power of the diet and insulin resistance.

Nonetheless, many studies are suggesting that the Alkaline diet can lower the risk of diabetes. Another devastating disease which alkaline diet helps getting rid of would be cancer. As you know, the Alkaline diet enables you to have a less hospitable environment for the cancer cells, which makes this diet an excellent idea for people who are looking to reduce this risk.

In regards to a healthier life, the Alkaline diet has also shown to reduce the risk of obesity. One study done on obese women suggested that alkaline diet reduced the risk of obesity in women, which makes sense as it helps you lose and manage body weight.

These facts about the Alkaline diet show you how the alkaline diet can help you get free of many diseases, and some have been backed up with detailed studies, whereas others are still being researched.

Nonetheless, you can't say that about other diets out there. The Alkaline diet will help you to get rid of many things and prevent you from further having any diseases. There is no better way of getting rid of illness or problems without the use of modern medicine, and this diet is so powerful that it will also boost your immune system which will help you avoid small issues like the common flu. All in all, there are many rejuvenating properties which come along with Alkaline diet, so don't overlook it and keep all the positives in mind before you look at the negatives.

Reduce Stress and Inflammation

The Alkaline diet has shown a significant reduction in inflammation. As you know, inflammation causes many chronic diseases such as Alzheimer's, dementia, obesity, diabetes, and much more. Now, there are many ways that the Alkaline diet helps you get rid of inflammation. The first one being autophagy, as you know alkaline diet helps you with cell rejuvenation cleans up itself by eating out the old self and rejuvenating them with the newer stronger ones. If your body does not regenerate itself with more new cells, the older ones have stayed for an extended period can cause inflammation.

Now that we've talked about many ways. Alkaline diet enables you to reduce inflammation; let's talk about how the alkaline diet can help you get rid of stress. You see, inflammation and stress go hand in hand. If you have high levels of inflammation, chances are your stress levels are going to be higher. Which means that if you lower your inflammation, you will reduce your stress levels, and as you know, this diet helps with better brain function. Alkaline diet enables you to send better signals to your brain, which would equal a better functioning brain.

When your mind is functioning at its absolute peak, your levels of stress drop down. Better brain function will also help you get rid of any stress you might be having and will give you overall better health can help you reduce weight. Overall, the health benefits you get from the alkaline diet will help you get rid of your stress or at least lower it. Which means, even if you are not facing any stress-related issues, the alkaline diet will help you have a better functioning brain and also help you get rid of any mental fog or stress you might be dealing. With that in mind, always make sure you consult a physician if you are noticing much more stress than you can handle, as it can be something severe and not fixable by the Alkaline diet.

Improved Insulin Sensitivity

As you know, the Alkaline diet helps you get more insulin sensitive, which allows you with many things. To understand it better, let me explain to you how insulin works. Every time you eat a meal, your insulin spikes up, then insulin is used to shuttle food either to muscle or your fat store.

When you have too much glycogen in your bloodstream, your body will send that energy to your fat stores. Whereas if you're insulin sensitive, your body will send the glycogen to muscle stores and will be used for energy. When you are insulin sensitive, you are more likely to use up all the glycogen from your food faster, and not requiring your glycogen to be converted into fats.

How Alkaline diet helps with curing insulin resistance is by using up all the glycogen stores, making your body use up fat stores and when you eat good food, it will use up all the glycogen and shuttle it straight to the muscle mass to be used for energy instead of being stored into fat. That is how the Alkaline diet helps you become more insulin sensitive; the benefits of being insulin sensitive are many. Once you become insulin-sensitive, you will notice more mental energy and less mental fog, and you will also see less fat being stored in your body which makes it ideal for people looking to lose fat and or gain muscle.

Being insulin sensitive will also help you gain more muscle since most of the energy will be sent out to your muscle stores. It will be used to build stronger muscles instead of storing it into fat. Being insulin sensitive is a must, as it will also help you get rid of possible diseases such as type 2 diabetes. All in all, the Alkaline diet helps you tremendously with insulin sensitively, which will overall help you live a healthier life.

Boost Immune System

There is a reason why having a healthy immune system is fundamental, as it will help you get less sick and be more "immune" to disease. The alkaline diet has shown to increase the immune system so we will talk about how it boosts the immune system. There was a study done on stem cells when it comes down to a diet individual; more specifically, they took a look at how the stem cells rejuvenated.

The study concluded that Alkaline diet depleted white blood cells, which is precisely what we want so our body can produce better and more efficient cells, which lead to more production of stem cells and lesser of white cells. Once you start to get rid of your old white blood cells, you will begin to produce new ones, which will overall help you recover faster. This study also found that there was a reduced amount of protein kinase A (PKA), which allows the stem cells to regenerate. If you have a lower amount of (PKA), this means that it will enable the cells to turn on the regeneration mode, which will allow them to create new cells.

As you know, the Alkaline diet has shown to reduce insulin levels, which is a great thing for someone looking to boost their immune system. There was a study done showing that high amounts of insulin levels, prevented "T" cells from doing its job effectively. The "T" cells are here to suppress inflammation and to fight off illness, "T" cells are most of the time responsible for getting rid of toxins which cause disease and inflammation. When your insulin levels are high, "T" cells are not performing at their highest potential, which causes our immune system to drop down.

When you are diet, there isn't a requirement for insulin spikes, which lets our body help the "T" cells work at a higher level and overall, boosting our immune system. Since you aren't eating foods which will spike your insulin a crazy amount, this will give your digestive system and organs a break. When you eat a big meal, around 70% of the blood and energy goes to your stomach to digest it. Which means when you are on a diet, you give your body a chance to recover. Everything is healing when you are on the Alkaline diet, which includes the digestive system. Meaning, your gut will be working a lot more effectively once you have given it some time to heal.

As you know, digestion plays a significant role in both our mental health and immune system, about 60% of our immune system is in our colon, which means when you are the diet, you are recovering your whole body and overall boosting your immune system. You will be doing yourself a great service if you can manage to boost your immune system, and with all the backed-up science showing how Alkaline diet can help you promote your immune system and reduce many other health problems, there is no reason not to start Alkaline diet as soon as possible.

More Energy and Muscle Mass Increased

Even if your goal isn't to put on more muscle, it is still good to have more muscle mass as it helps you with many things. However, the main thing having higher amounts of muscle mass helps you with would be a fat loss; having a higher muscle mass will help you burn more fat since it increases your metabolic rate. Don't worry, and you don't have to look like a bodybuilder for that to happen; nonetheless, it is essential to have the right amount of muscle mass, especially for women.

The Alkaline diet has shown to increase and preserve muscle mass, so let's talk about how that happens. There was a study done between two groups of men, one followed an 80/20 diet method, and the other followed a healthy eating pattern. Both groups followed the same workout but a different diet, one group which supported the 80/20 diet, which we will talk about later in this book, they noticed after eight weeks was, both the groups gained and preserved the same amount of muscle, but the group who were following the Alkaline diet lost more fat.

This shows that the Alkaline diet not only helped followers gain muscle and preserve it, but it also helped them lose fat simultaneously. The main reason behind that is growth hormone, as you know, the Alkaline diet has shown to increase growth hormone in our bodies. What growth hormone mainly does, it allows a lot less muscle breakdown and to burn more fat, which is one of the primary reasons why the Alkaline diet is so beneficial for building and preserving muscle mass.

Another great benefit of the Alkaline diet as you know is higher energy levels, and there is a reason behind it. Many people know how it feels to have a sugar crash, you feel tired and lethargic, and the culprit behind it is insulin. When insulin is spiked up, your energy level goes down as this gives your brain a signal to relax. When you are an Alkaline diet, there are no insulin spikes throughout the day, which provides you with more energy.

Another reason why you have more energy when you are diet is that your body goes into a fight or flight response and since your body is eating food it was intended to eat in the first place, and our body produces more adrenaline throughout the day, which gives you more energy as you go along. Just be aware, at the beginning of your diet journey, you might feel less energized.

The reason behind it is because your body is still getting used to these changes, but after a week or two, you should start to notice more energy. Use the power to get more work done at work and gym. In my opinion, and this is the most significant benefit which comes along with the Alkaline diet. More energy makes you feel a lot better when you are looking towards making it thru those long days.

These are all the main benefits which come along when you start the diet, and the benefits genuinely outweigh all the negatives which might happen. These benefits can be life changing to most people, lowering the risk of diseases and increasing longevity it's a fantastic thing to have. Alkaline diet provides you with that and then some.

Chapter 3: What Is pH Level and How to Measure Them

Now that we have discussed the benefits which come along the alkaline diet, and also what the alkaline diet is. Let's talk about the next major issue, which would be the pH level. When following the alkaline diet, it is imperative that you have a clear idea of what the pH level is and what it calls for. Understanding how to test out your pH level, is very crucial when following the alkaline diet, especially in the beginning. To help you understand what pH level is, it is essentially a way to test out how acidic or alkaline you are. As mentioned previously, the scale goes from 1 to 14. If your pH level is at 1, then there's a high chance that you are extremely acidic. Whereas if your pH level goes to 14, that just means you are very alkaline. Ideally, you want to be somewhere around 7.5 pH to see optimal results. Even when you are following the alkaline diet, you don't want to be in the extreme ends of either way. Meaning, it isn't always the best idea to be extremely alkaline.

With that in mind, always remember to aim for a middle point in the pH level, which is 7.5. Your pH level will fluctuate throughout the day, which is totally fine. However, if your average is at 7.5 pH throughout the whole day, then you should be totally fine and be at an alkaline state overall.

That being said, there are many ways to test your pH levels. The main two tests would be the saliva pH and the urine pH. Many people don't know this, but these two tests are very different from one another. One will be a lot more acidic, whereas the other one won't be as acidic when compared, which is why it is essential that you understand the difference between the two methods and how you should use them accordingly based on your goals. The first thing you need to understand when it comes to pH levels is that the saliva will always be higher at the alkaline level. Depending on your diet, your saliva will be more readily available to see where your pH level is, based on the foods which you ate.

This will factor in the food you have eaten and how you have digested the food. One of the things you need to keep in mind when checking your saliva is that if you have eaten anything which is very Alkaline. If so, then it will show that your body is an Alkaline state, even if it isn't. This could be misleading when trying to find out if your body is alkaline, which is why many people recommend testing your pH level 30 to 40 minutes after you have eaten, especially when testing the saliva. Most of the time, your saliva will be the most accurate test when done correctly. Unlike your urine, your urine will be a lot more acidic naturally and will be less alkaline when it comes to testing your pH levels. There's a reason to that, the main reason why the alkaline levels will be a lot lower when testing out your urine is for a straightforward reason which is that your urine typically gets rid of toxins in your body. Especially in the morning when you wake up, and you haven't urinated in a long time, your body will be cleaning out all your organs and pissing out all the toxins which are available in your body, which is why your urine will always be a lot more acidic level when compared to your saliva. Now when people are following the Alkaline diet, most of the time, they test both the urine level pH and their saliva level pH to get a better understanding of their body. You have to understand, when you are urinating, you are getting rid of toxins, which are most of the time very acidic.

Which is why you need to understand how to read your urine samples accordingly, your urine also contains a lot of sodium and waste products from all your organs, which is why specialist measure the pH level differently. The average pH level in urine is 6 pH; anything under 5 will be considered acidic. However, anything higher than 8 is alkaline. The same thing goes for the saliva pH levels; your level will fluctuate on how much food you're eating and what kind of foods you might have consumed recently. For example, a high protein meal before you test your pH level using the urine test will lead to a higher acidic level, which is why we recommend you wait it out. However, if you have a high alkaline level reading from your urine, there's a high chance that you might have thrown up a lot or you might have urinary tract infection. It is not ideal for you to be entirely alkaline when it comes to following this diet. If you are at the higher side of being alkaline from your urine test, then this could be not a good sign. You have to understand that you cannot be overly acidic or overly alkaline. Ideally, you want to be more on the alkaline side, which is why you need to be eating more alkaline foods to see better results as previously mentioned. However, your urine will always be on the acidic side, so be aware of that once you start following this diet. In fact, the water you drink is also going to dictate how acidic you are once you start following this diet.

Also, the pH level in the urine can vary differently. Many doctors don't even use urine pH level test your pH levels anymore as it is so unreliable. The doctors will only use the urine pH level to understand more information if needed, which is why we recommend that you don't use it either. However, if you're still stern on using this method, then there's a specific kit which you can get from any drugstore which will let you urinate in a box, and will test out your pH level accordingly. Since there a lot of methods to test it out, we're not going to get into all the ways of testing out your urine samples and your pH levels. Just make sure that you go to the drug store and figure out which one you want to go with, and then follow the instructions on the box.

This is if you actually want to test your pH level using the urine samples, if you are eating a right amount of alkaline food then there are no worries when it comes to testing out urine levels and your pH levels overall. On the other hand, the spit or saliva pH level can be beneficial. When it comes to testing out your saliva levels of pH level, it is imperative that you understand how to use it properly and how to get the best results out of it. You have to realize that the saliva level will be a lot more accurate when it comes to testing out your pH level, as we told you previously saliva does not hold any of the toxicity which urine does. Most of the time, saliva gives you a better understanding of where your pH level is throughout the whole diet.

Your pH level should be around 6 to 8 when you're testing out your saliva levels. Ideally, your pH level should be at 7.5 as this will give you the best results. This is one of the best areas to be in when it comes to being alkaline. To test out, your saliva level it is very straightforward, simply go to your nearest drug store and get those strips which will allow you to get your pH level reading. The first thing you need to do is take the colored part on top off the strip and put it underneath your tongue, making sure you get enough saliva on it. Once you've gotten enough saliva in the strip then take it out after 30 seconds of putting it in your mouth and shake it up, it will give you a color scheme which will provide you with an idea where your pH level is. On the box of the strips, it will have the color scheme which will show you where your pH level stands.

If you have ever used keto strips, then you will feel at home using the pH strips. Instead, it will test out your pH levels. One thing to make sure when you start your test of pH levels using your saliva is to make sure that you haven't eaten or drunk any alkaline water before you test it. Give yourself at least 30 to 40 minutes before you start to use the pH strip to see where your pH level is, as we previously told you whatever you eat will show up on the pH test.

Which is something you don't want; we want to understand where your pH levels are at naturally in our body and not by the foods that we just recently ate. We know that the specific foods that we're going to be eating to alkalize your body are essential, however, once you do eat those alkaline foods, it will give you an unauthentic pH level reading. This sometimes happens after eating alkaline food, and your pH level tends to show up around 8 or 9, this would not be an accurate reading. Make sure when you do test out your pH level that it is correctly scheduled, and you haven't eaten in about 30 to 40 minutes this will give you the best reading when it comes to pH level reading overall.

Now, the ideal urine and saliva pH sample should be around 7.2 when factored in both of their results. If you do both a urine sample and a saliva sample, and the average of both is 7.2 ph, then you are it the perfect spot. If your saliva sample goes below 7, then there's a high chance of your body starting to become acidic, add more alkaline foods which will allow you to become less acidic hence making you more alkaline. The recommended times you should be checking your pH level varies from person to person, and some people will say that you should check your pH level every two to three times a day.

However, some people recommend that you only need to check your pH level two to three times a week. We have found that the best schedule would be to test your pH level once a day, depending on how acidic or alkaline you are you might need to monitor it more frequently. The best way to go about testing your pH level would be to monitor it once a day. However, if you are more acidic and you're looking to become alkaline very quickly then we recommend that you check your saliva pH level two to three times a day to see where your levels are at for a week or two. Once you've achieved a right balance of pH levels, then it will be time to let it rest and then check your pH level less frequently allowing you to save money on strips and have a better idea on where your pH levels are.

Once you become alkaline and your body becomes more alkalized the chances of becoming acidic you are will drop. You see when you're more alkaline, your insulin levels will drop, your inflammation levels will fall, and you will notice less pain overall. Once you become more acidic, your digestion will slow down, and you will feel more pain, and your inflammation will go up. These are a great sign to see when you are acidic or when you are alkaline. Understand your body will give you signs, which is why we highly recommend you start understanding how your body functions when it is acidic and when it is alkaline. Just so you can understand a little bit better, the first thing you need to do is understand that the urine sample is to be you are used on a rare occasion or if you want to be extra meticulous with your pH level. Many doctors don't even recommend that you use urine to test out your pH level overall, as urine levels can be very unreliable when it comes to testing out your pH levels. Your saliva pH levels will be a lot more accurate, for the average person to test on how acidic or alkaline you are. If you are to test your saliva and your urine pH levels, then make sure that your pH level is at 7.2 which will make it the ideal pH level overall when it comes to making sure that you are at the alkaline side of the body.

As always, when you're testing your urine pH level that you test it after you have done urinating first thing in the morning, ideally midday when you have drunk enough water and your liver and other organs have been cleaned up. On the other hand, your saliva test should not be done once you have eaten anything, ideally. Wait for 30 to 40 minutes before you test your pH level after you're done eating food, as this could give you a wrong reading once you have eaten a portion of food and test your pH level right after.

The foods can dictate how your pH levels going to be, which is why it is ideal that you wait down a bit before you test out your pH levels. Furthermore, depending on your acidic levels, you also need to understand how your body functions when it is a lot more acidic, and when it is more alkaline. That way, you don't have to keep testing your pH levels, as you can tell by the way your body is performing to get a better idea of your acidic or alkaline levels. If you do eat alkaline or acidic food, make sure to counteract it by eating a different type of food to make sure that your pH level is balanced. With that in mind, now you've got a good idea on how to test your pH levels and the different types of pH levels when it comes to you being alkaline and acidic overall. You can now utilize the right methods, which you think will benefit you greatly, after reading this chapter. Make sure that you don't spend too much money on pH level strips, as it is essential that you don't take this very seriously. In the beginning, it is ideal that you test your ph levels regularly. However, once you have gotten the idea of how your body feels when it is acidic or alkaline, then you will not have to check it so frequently.

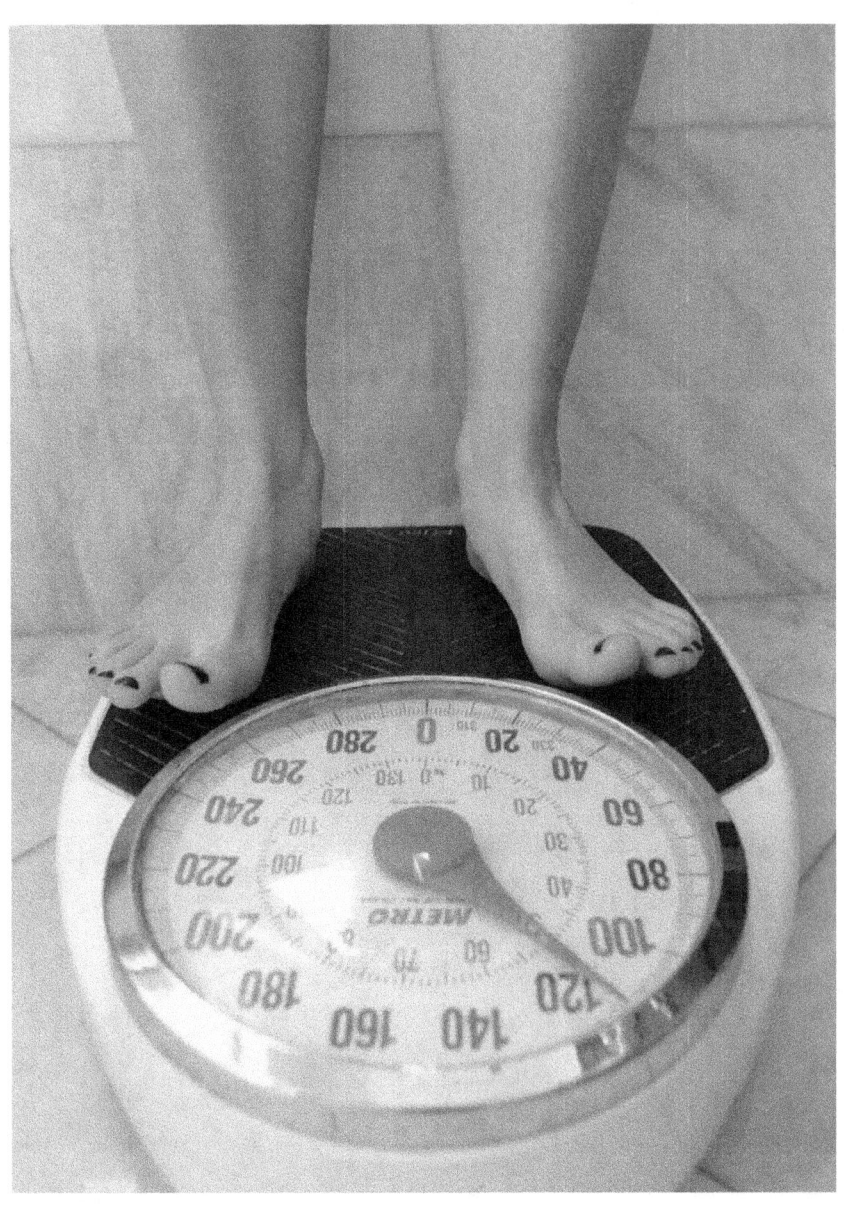

Chapter 4: Macronutrients

When you are following the alkaline diet, it is essential that you take care of your macronutrient needs, which is why in this chapter, we are going to be talking about the macronutrient requirements when following the alkaline diet. The one thing you have to keep in mind when following the alkaline diet is that the number of macronutrients you're getting into your body can dictate how acidic or alkaline you're going to be, which is why it is imperative that you pick out the macronutrient needs appropriately, and of course, based on your goals. Many of you have a goal of getting rid of diseases, or to just stay healthy overall. Which is great but one thing you have to keep in mind is that when following the alkaline diet is that you cannot have too much protein as it can become very acidic, on the other hand, you can't have zero protein since protein is a requirement for your daily needs. It doesn't matter if you want to put on muscle or just to stay healthy, you need protein in your diet, which is why you can't get rid of it completely.

As you know, when following the alkaline diet, you are a vegan. Since you're not allowed to have any meat, you're going to have to resort to vegan protein to keep your body as alkaline as possible. When you are a vegan, the chances of you having too many carbs in your diet will go up tremendously. The reason why it will go up is that most of the foods that come from plants tend to be higher in the carbohydrates department. Which is why you need to make sure whatever it is that you're doing you are keeping your carbohydrates in control when following the alkaline diet. You also have to take into consideration the number of fats you're going to be consuming when following the alkaline diet, it is more so important that you get enough fats in your diet since it will help you with your bodily function and your hormone production. If you didn't know this, the amount of fats you get into your body is very crucial, and it is perhaps the most essential macronutrient you can get into your body.

Our body produces hormones and other things thanks to the number of fats we're going to be consuming, which means you cannot neglect the amount of fat you are to be eating when following the alkaline diet. With that being said, you have to keep in mind that your macronutrient ratio will be a lot different depending on your goal. We are going to talk about all three goals which many people would be striving towards when following the alkaline diet. Most of the time, people following the alkaline diet are either looking to lose weight, be healthy overall, and not attract any diseases and finally to get rid of any diseases that they might be facing. But that being said, let's talk about the three goals and how to achieve it with managing your macronutrient needs.

Lose Weight

If you are someone looking to lose weight, then the alkaline diet could definitely work for you. However, making sure that you get enough macronutrients in your diet can be a bit difficult. With that being said, let's talk about the macronutrient needs you will be required when following the alkaline diet. Keep in mind that you will not be getting enough protein if you don't take care of it. Meaning, you have to be extra meticulous with the foods that you're eating in order to get enough protein in your diet. Achieving weight loss with the alkaline diet could happen, but you also have to make sure that you're getting enough exercise in your daily routine to supplement your goals. We'll talk about workout routine later on in the book but keep in mind that for you to achieve the weight loss, you will have to get some physical activity. Now the ideal macronutrient breakdown would be 40% protein, 40% carbs and 20% fat; this would give you a perfect macronutrient balance that will help you to lose body fat and to get enough protein in your diet. Keep in mind that when your goal is to lose weight, you need to make sure that your protein is on the higher side. The reason why your protein needs to be on the higher side is that protein takes the most calories to digest, which means you will burn calories only by eating protein.

It doesn't matter where you get your protein from; you will still be burning a lot of calories simply by digesting the amount of protein that you're eating. Having a 40% carb ratio is an excellent place to be in when your goal is to lose body fat, especially when you have accompanied it with a good workout plan, you will need some energy to get through those workouts. Which is why quickly available energy is very important in the form of carbs, the carbs will definitely help you to get through your workouts and your daily needs, whether you work or daily chores, which is why we kept the carbohydrates on the higher side. Now with the fat, you need to make sure that you are getting at least 20% fats in your diet for optimal hormone production and overall well-being. If your hormones are out of whack, then there's a chance that you will not be burning as much body fat as you would like to.

Which is why it is essential that you make sure you are getting enough fats in your daily diet. The amount of fat will definitely help you with the energy, and also to keep your hormones at optimal levels so that you can actually burn fat. Finally, when you are looking towards losing weight, make sure that your calories are below your maintenance. Which means, if you need 2000 calories to maintain your body weight, then make sure that you are only eating 1800 calories. Now this book isn't about macronutrients entirely, but this just gives you a brief an example of how many calories you would need to lose weight. Figure out how many calories you need to maintain your body weight and take off 200 calories. This will give you a great spot to be in, in terms of losing body weight and to achieve the goal that you're going towards.

Lower the Risk of Diseases

When your goal is to lower the number of illnesses which you might attract, you have to take into consideration that you have to be more on the alkaline side in order to achieve this goal. Which would mean that you cannot have as much protein as someone who is merely looking to lose weight. That being said, let's talk about the macronutrient needs you will be required when your goal is to lower the risk of diseases and to see better results overall. The first thing you have to make sure when following the alkaline diet is that you need to start by eating the right foods that will allow you to stay alkaline. You will have to be a little more meticulous with the amount and the types of food that you're going to be eating when your goal is mainly to lower the risk of diseases. Which means, the chances of you slipping up and having something more on the acidic side should be slim to none.

Moreover, you also need to test your acidic levels more frequently, especially in the beginning, to make sure that you are on the alkaline side. That being said, let's talk about the macronutrient, which would be ideal for someone who's looking to lower the risk of diseases. The perfect macronutrient breakdown would be 30% protein 50% carbs and 20% fats. The reason why the protein is on the lower side when compared to someone who's looking to lose weight is that having higher protein can make you more acidic. Our goal is to make sure that you are not on the acidic side based on your goal. Also, we need to make sure that you are not overexerting your body by eating tons of protein.

As you know, protein takes a lot of energy to digest the food, which is why a decent amount of protein in your diet which will help you to maintain the muscle mass that you have while keeping the body very alkaline. At this point, you can also consider having alkaline water to enhance your levels of alkaline throughout the day further. Now when you are looking towards reducing the risk of diseases, you can still have the calories that you want. But ideally, you should not go over the maintenance calories that you need throughout the day if you overate then chances of you putting on more weight will go up and therefore increase the risk of diseases. Only half the number of calories you need to maintain your body weight and go from there, if you follow this method, then you should be at a better position of lowering the risk of diseases.

Get Rid of Diseases

Now if you're at an unfortunate situation where you are facing diseases, then there is still hope for you. There have been many personal experiences showing that the alkaline diet has helped users to get rid of cancer, and to help them with chemotherapy. Moreover, if you're facing hypertension or any other diseases, the alkaline diet can genuinely help you to get rid of those. Keep in mind that these claims came through personal experiences and that this has not been backed up by science. However, since many people are claiming that they have gotten rid of diseases using the alkaline diet, then you might as well try it. Now when your goal is to get rid of diseases the macronutrient breakdown is going to be a little bit more different than both of these diets, the ideal macronutrient breakdown for you getting rid of diseases would be 20% protein, 50% carbs, and 30% fats.

This would be the complete breakdown for someone who's looking to get rid of their diseases, keep in mind that 20% protein will just give you enough protein to maintain your muscle mass. Our goal is to stay as alkaline is possible to get rid of the diseases, which is why we're taking the bare minimum amount of protein throughout the day to ensure that we are keeping our muscles intact and that we are strong. Staying strong when you have diseases, is very crucial when it comes to seeing better results overall. But that being said, the reason why the protein is so low is simply that to keep our body very alkaline and to see the most results out of this diet.

On the other hand, the carbohydrates are similar to someone who's looking to reduce the risk of diseases. The carbs aren't so crucial as they are simply just energy sources, and 50% carbs are wonderful when your goal is to get rid of your disease and stay healthy overall. The amount of fat that we're going to be eating it's going to be a little bit higher when compared to other methods, our fat is going to be 30%. The reason why 30% is because for you to see better results with your hormone production. It is essential that you take care of your hormone imbalances when you are facing diseases, which is why we kept a fat a little bit higher for our body to have enough fat so we can use it as energy and hormone production benefits.

Keep in mind that the fat is actually used as energy similar to carbs. However, it takes longer to convert into energy, whereas carbohydrates are more readily available for you to use up as energy. Which is why it is essential that you understand this and take care of your carbs and fats accordingly, and to use them for energy benefits. One thing you have to make sure when following the diet, especially when your goal to get rid of diseases, is to make sure that you're drinking alkaline water. Having alkaline water would be very important when your goal is to get rid of diseases such as cancer, this will give you that extra oomph that you're looking for when it comes to getting rid of those diseases. That being said, you also have to take into consideration that you have to keep checking your alkaline levels throughout the whole day to see if you are on the alkaline side. In terms of the calories you need throughout the day, you will just need the maintenance calories based on your body weight.

If you are going through chemotherapy, then your bodyweight will definitely fluctuate, so adjust your calories accordingly. Now, as always consult with your doctor or physician before you start any diet, especially when you are facing diseases. This is just personal experience from many people, and we are sharing it with you, by no means, the diet can scientifically help you get rid of your diseases although it has helped many people.

Why Are Macronutrients so Important

Regardless of you following the alkaline diet or not, having the right number of macronutrients in your daily food intake is very important. Understanding how many calories you need and the protein carbs and fats, which will help you achieve your goal. Keep in mind that everybody's nutrient needs are going to be completely different, and therefore we have broken down the macronutrient needs much as we can to help people understand. With that in mind, you also need to understand that when you are following the alkaline diet, you should never go over 40% of your calories coming from protein. This is for a straightforward reason; the reason is that if you have too much protein, then you will simply be acidic. You will never achieve the real alkaline state that you're looking for if you have way too much protein in your diet, and most of the time people think they do need a lot of protein, thanks to the false information that has been provided to you online. Sure, if you're a competitive bodybuilder, then you most definitely need a higher amount of protein, however competitive bodybuilders are not looking towards becoming alkaline they are merely looking towards putting on as much muscle as possible. Which is why they might need the high protein, whereas if you're just an average Joe who works out here and there, then you definitely do not need more than 40% of the calories coming from protein. You will still put on muscle by eating 40% of the calories come from protein, don't think that you need a lot of protein for you to achieve your goals. If you do have a lot of protein, then you will be a lot more in the acidic and therefore not be following the alkaline diet. When you think about it, in order for you to be on the alkaline side, you definitely should be eating a moderate amount of protein but not too extreme. Which is why it is essential to understand your macronutrients need especially when you're following the alkaline diet, luckily the carbohydrates in the fat do not play a significant role in terms of making you more acidic or alkaline. Which is why it is essential that you take care of the situation as much as possible by eating less protein. We can't stress enough how protein can make you acidic, which is why you need to consider this and rectified as soon as possible if eating a lot of protein especially when you follow the alkaline diet. Luckily when you are following the alkaline diet, then you will be getting most of your protein thru vegan sources. Naturally, your intake of protein is going to go down and therefore help you achieve that alkalinity that you are looking for. However, keep in mind that you do not go over 40% of your calories coming from protein.

With that being said, we come to the conclusion of this chapter. Thank you so much for sticking around through this whole chapter, and we hope that you learned a lot from it. Make sure that your macros are taken care of after reading this chapter. It is essential that you take care of it, as a place of large roll on how acidic or alkaline you are to be. With that being said, read this chapter very carefully and understand how to take care of your needs.

Chapter 5: Good and Bad Foods

Even if you don't understand how most diets work, you know that processed meats are very bad for you when it comes to health and wellness. There have been many studies showing that process meat can cause many diseases and illness. Moreover, they happen to be backed up with detailed studies to prove as such. When following the alkaline diet, you are not allowed to eat any processed meat, which makes this diet one of the better diets when it comes to living a healthier life. As we explained to you in the previous chapters, all the benefits of alkaline diet you, can now see how it can be an excellent idea for you to start following this diet.

With that being said, let's talk about some of the negatives you might face when eating processed meats. That way, you can understand how and when to cut it out and give you more of an incentive to start following the alkaline diet. For people that don't know what processed meat is, it is mostly meat that has been preserved by curing, salting, smoking, drying, and canning. So the foods that are considered to be processed meats are, sausage, hot dog, salami, hams, salted, cured meat smoked meat, dried meat, beef jerky, canned tuna Etc. As you can tell, especially in the European and North American regions of the world we can see a lot of these foods consumed.

Which is why they face more adversities when it comes to diseases in those specific areas. If you live in North America or a European country, then you will be facing a lot more of these diseases and problems. One of the most important things when it comes to eating processed meat is that it has been linked to an unhealthy lifestyle. Processed meat has been associated with being around people who are living an unhealthy life overall. Also, as you know, many people in the United States tend to live an unhealthy lifestyle and eat a ton of processed food. One example would be that many people who smoke cigarettes tend to eat a lot of processed meats.

Also, people who drink much alcohol will consume a lot of processed meat when they are intoxicated. This is a prevalent practice, which makes it a very unhealthy lifestyle decision. Ask yourself, when was the last time you consumed processed meat, there is a high chance that you were intoxicated the last time you consumed processed meat. Most of the time, you are eating processed meats when you are intoxicated or smoking a lot of cigarettes. Moreover, people who eat a lot of processed meat tend to consume fewer fruits and vegetables.

If you're not eating the right amount of fiber and micronutrients in your diet, then there's a high chance that you're not living a healthy life overall. Basically, people who are not living a healthy life tend to consume a lot of processed meats. If you're one of them, then make sure that you rectify this situation as quickly as possible by cutting out the unhealthy things in your life which includes processed meat. Another thing that processed meat has been linked with would be chronic diseases. Eating processed meat can increase the risk of high blood pressure, heart diseases, cancer, and chronic obstructive pulmonary disease. There have been many studies showing, the people who eat this kind of meats tend to have a higher chance of attracting diseases stated above. There have also been studies done on an animal which has been consuming processed meat, and it showed that their cancer risk where bought higher when consuming processed meat as compared to when there were not.

The reason why is because processed meat contains harmful chemicals that may increase the risk of chronic diseases. There are numerous chemicals in processed meat; one of them is nitrite. This compound is one of the main reasons why your risk of cancer increases when consuming processed meat. The reason why the use of the compound is to preserve the red, pink color of the meat. To also improve the taste of the meat and finally to get rid of any bacteria or growth in the long-term. Another reason why process meat cannot be right for you is that it has been smoked. As we know, meat smoking is widespread when it comes to preservation.

It has often been salted and dried, to extend the shelf life of it. Once you get smoke meat in a burning wood and charcoal with dripping fat burns on a hot surface, it can cause many chemicals to form in the heat and hence making the meat very unhealthy. Which is why it isn't a good idea to consume processed meats in the long-term, the way it has been made and processed makes it a terrible idea for you to consume it. There was one study done that showed when consuming processed meat every day equals to smoking ten cigarettes a day in regards to the health affects you might face when consuming processed meat. Which goes to show how bad processed meat can be for you. Another thing is that processed meat contains trans-fat. As you know trans-fat is a human-made fat which has been causing many side effects in our health and wellness.

A decent amount of good fats in our diet is significant for optimal hormone production, etc. However, trans-fat can be very bad for us in the long term as a can cause many problems. One of the issues you might face when consuming trans-fat is the lowered amount of good cholesterol and the increase of bad cholesterol. Also, processed meat contains a lot of sodium, which can be very bad for us in the long-term. As you know, high amounts of sodium consumption can cause many illnesses and diseases. One of the significant things that it can cause is the risk of high blood pressure. High amounts of sodium have shown to increase blood pressure and inflammation increase, which is why it is not advisable for people to eat a lot of sodium when consuming processed meat. Processed meat can cause a lot of issues as we know by now, but one of the significant things that have been found in the recent studies is there is an increased risk of breast cancer.

There were one study shows, that when women consumed processed meat such as hot dogs, the risk of breast cancer went up 9%. Which isn't high when you think about it, but why have that issue when it can be avoided. Overall, the risk of type 2 diabetes will go up 19% and the risk of heart disease while going up to 42% when consuming processed meat. These studies have been backed up by proper scientific studies done in a lab, which goes to show that processed meat cannot be good for health and overall well-being, which is one of the reasons why the alkaline diet does not allow you to eat meat in general, as a meat has been shown to increase the acidic levels in your body. The whole premise behind the alkaline diet is that you are not to consume foods which will raise your acidic level in your body when you have high acidic levels in your body, and there's a high chance for you to consume more bacteria. When there are more bacteria in your body, there's a high chance for you to attract more diseases and illness.

When it comes to attracting disease growing in your body, the bacteria like the acidic environment of your body, hence, when your body is sick, you will attract more of those diseases, and it will be more likely for you to grow them when your body is acidic. One of the most acidic things you can consume would be the use of processed meats. As you know, the processed meats can cause many issues, as stated in this chapter above. If you're looking to follow the alkaline diet and then there's no chance in hell that you're going to be eating any processed meat. Even if you're someone looking to better your health, the first thing you need to do is cut out any process me that you are going to be having in your meats.

We can tell you what you should do and should not do, but as you can tell by the evidence that processed meat is not the answer when it comes to living a healthier life. More often than not, many of your consuming process meat and you don't even know it. Did you know that meats that are not organic and have been cut mechanically, are also considered processed meats? These meats have been cut in a way which can cause many issues. Unfortunately, our system has made everything unhealthy when it comes to consuming food.

Which is why as a consumer we need to be very smart with the foods that we're going to be eating, which means that any meat is not a good idea for us in this day and age? The reason why is because we can't trust any meat and how it is coming to us. Back in the 1940s, we would be able to butcher our meat and understand where it is coming from. However, now, it is impossible. First, understand where this meat is coming from how healthy the animal was and what kind of hormones they have been given. Also, if you didn't know, many animals have been pumped with unhealthy hormones to produce more meat in them, allowing them to make more money for the meat producers, which is why the alkaline diet is one of the best options when it comes to bettering yourself and to live a healthier life. As Alkaline diet cuts out any foods that we have no idea about if you don't know where it came from that there's a high chance that you're not eating it.

Also, alkaline diet only allows you to eat alkaline foods, and you do not consume any foods which will raise your acidic levels in your body. When your alkaline, you will be a lot healthier as you will notice once you start following the diet. However, the main take-home message from this chapter is the importance of not consuming process meat or any meat in general. In this day and age, there are many chemicals put on to the meat. Even the meats that are considered processed are processed, which means that there's no chance that you are getting good quality meat when you're consuming any types of food. The next time you see any processed meat, make sure to throw it out and start consuming better foods for yourself if your goal is to live a healthier life.

When you're following the alkaline diet, you will not be allowed to eat any meat. As you can see in this chapter above, eating meat can be very unhealthy for you since you don't know where the meat is coming from and how it is processed. The foods that you can eat when following the alkaline diet are mostly fruits and vegetables. Even then, there are certain fruits and vegetables that you can and cannot eat. We will give you a full chart showcasing what types of fruits and vegetables you can and cannot eat, overall you need to understand that eating fruits and vegetables at the right amount. That is very crucial when following the alkaline diet. Now to give you an idea of the that you can eat when following the alkaline diet would be fruits, vegetables, seeds, legumes, and tofu. This gives you a brief idea on the food, so you know which ones you can eat, you should already know the food so you should stay away from which would be dairy, coffee, alcohol, fish, meat, any processed foods. Even when you are eating particular fruit and vegetable, you still need to see how acidic it is. Evidently enough, there are some very acidic fruits, and therefore, you need to stay away from. Here's what we're going to do, we're going to give you a chart of foods which will show you foods which are alkaline and acidic. That way, you can have a great Idea on what you can and cannot eat.

Highly Alkaline food	Alkaline food	Acidic food
Broccoli	Beetroot	Processed meat
Cucumber	Cabbage	Milk
Celery	Cauliflower	Apple
Kale	Tomato	Tropical fruits
Asparagus	Coconut oil	Eggs
Spinach	Coconut	Raisins
Parsley	Zucchini	Cranberries
Sprouts	Artichokes	Grapes
Green Drinks	Brussels sprouts	Dates
Grasses	Himalayan salt	Mango

As you can see by the foods listed above, there are many foods which we would consider to be healthy but are on the acidic side. This chart will give you a great idea on foods which you should and should not eat when following the alkaline diet. Keep in mind, there is a ton of different foods in this world, if we had to make a chart showing all the foods, then it would take up the whole book. Nonetheless, pick your meals accordingly after going thru this chart. This chart will overall make you more self-efficient when it comes to eating the right food when following the alkaline diet.

By now, you should have a clear idea of what the alkaline diet is, which means you have an idea on what the Alkaline water is and what the water can do in terms of benefits and making you more alkaline overall. Many people say that the Alkaline water can help you regulate your body's pH level, and prevent many diseases, including cancer. What is alkaline water, exactly? And why is it essential when it comes to following the alkaline diet and getting better results overall. The alkaline water refers to its pH level, as you know, the pH level measure is how acidic or alkaline you are or the food. The scale ranges from 0 to 14, one being very acidic and 13 being very alkaline as we told you in the previous chapters with the sweet spot at 7.5 pH.

Simply put, the Alkaline water has a higher level of pH level, which will help your body to become more alkaline, increasing your alkaline level and will neutralize your acidic level in the body. Which is why many people recommend that you drink alkaline water, right after you drink or eat something which is highly acidic to counteract the balance issue and to alkalize your body overall. Fresh drinking water is generally around 7, whereas the alkaline water is typically about 8 or 9 ph. However, the pH level isn't the most important things when it comes to making alkaline water. The Alkaline water must contain alkaline minerals which will allow it to have higher antioxidants. Hence making it more alkaline and change to your body in a better way when it comes to alkalizing your body.

It isn't always necessary that the water should be higher in the alkaline level, it is essential that you make sure that your alkaline body is absorbing the minerals and making it more alkaline. Hopefully, that makes sense, make sure that your body is alkaline not because of the alkaline level in the food or drinks, but it is alkaline from the inside. Although there have not been any studies showing that the alkaline diet can be right for you when it comes to making your body more alkaline, there have been some people saying that the alkaline water could make you get rid of many diseases even if you're not following the alkaline diet.

As you guys might know the tap water is not the safest when it comes to drinking, which is why many people who aren't following the alkaline diet and start drinking alkaline water tend to notice better health benefits because there aren't any added chemicals to it. Our tap water can be very polluted, which is why many people resort to bottled water or more accurately, alkaline water these days to see better health benefits.

Had our tap water been less polluted, we would not be drinking alkaline water to see better results. Just for reference, the tap water is around 7 pH or close to 7 pH whereas the alkaline water has to be above 7 pH for to be called the alkaline water. Our bodies do a fantastic job of maintaining blood pH level, which is why it is not recommended by many people to start drinking alkaline water to see better results.

Nonetheless, alkaline water can help you alkalize your body quickly when compared to drinking regular tap water. If your goal is to become alkaline very quickly, alkaline water can help you tremendously as it is already alkalized and therefore will make your body more alkaline throughout the whole day once you start drinking it as we told you previously, if your very acidic, alkaline water can definitely help you become more alkaline. However, if you're not following the alkaline diet then it will be tough for you to become alkaline overall even if you are drinking alkaline water, so think of the alkaline water more as a supplement to your diet. Sure, the alkaline water will make you more alkaline to a certain degree, but it won't turn you into an alkaline body overall if you're not following the alkaline diet.

Alkaline water is not great just for the alkaline level, and it is even better because of the mineral contents in it. As you know, the tap water does not have as many minerals as we think it does, more specifically, it isn't as clean and is less polluted when compared to alkaline water, which is why most people tend to drink alkaline water, to see better results and to get more gains out of it. But once you do start drinking the alkaline water make sure that you are drinking it for the right reasons and that you don't have any health conditions, many people who do have kidney conditions or are taking medications to alter the kidney function it can be harmful to them.

Some of the minerals in alkaline water, cannot be healthy for most people if they are taking any medications or are working on some kidney rehab. Which is why it is essential that you ask your doctor before you start drinking alkaline water regularly, you see our body is not accustomed to alkaline water before we start drinking. Unfortunately, we are accustomed to tap water or the normal water as we get in our country, which is why alkaline water needs to be assessed before you start drinking it for the right reasons. If your healthy male or female then you should have no problem with alkaline water as you'll see significant benefits out of it, however, if you are taking any medications or under supervision make sure you consult with your doctor before you start drinking the alkaline water.

Since you have now understood the function of the alkaline water and how can help you accordingly, let's talk about some of the benefits that you might see from drinking alkalized water. One of the benefits that you will see from drinking alkaline water is the reduced risk of chronic diseases, more specifically, chronic acidosis. If you have a low-grade chronic acidosis then it might help you that you start drinking some of the alkalized water, the study has not been concrete yet, but there is some suggestion showing that it will help you. Another thing the alkaline water helps you with is to help you with improving your overall health.

As we know by now alkalizing your body will help you with better bodily functions, better digestion, etc. Which is why many people recommend they start drinking alkaline water to better yourself, however, you have to remember that if you want to see better results, then you need to make sure that you are following the alkaline diet alongside with the

consumption of your alkalized water. In fact, many people who are facing certain conditions should avoid excessive mineral intake, as mentioned to you previously if you have any kidney conditions, then you need to make sure they consult with your doctor before you start drinking any alkaline water. Another thing that the alkaline water can help you with is to improved athletic performance, again this study has not been concrete yet, but many athletes are suggesting that alkalize water has helped them perform for a more extended period at their peak performance. If you're an athlete, then try out the alkaline water and see how it does for you.

Many people suggest that it will help you. However, many athletes say that it does not help them overall whereas some do say so, it is a gray matter and therefore needs to be found out by the person itself. Finally, there have been many studies showing that alkaline water can help you with digestion health. This is a great study, but it is up in the air when it comes to the alkalized water helping you with digestion. As we told you previously when you're alkaline, your body will digest food a lot better, which is why many people start on the alkaline diet. So it just makes sense if you are drinking alkalized water, that you will see better digestion health overall. Now, that you're aware of the alkaline water and how to use it properly let's talk about how to acquire alkaline water for the best results possible. One of the things you need to understand is that the alkaline water can be very expensive once you start drinking it regularly, which is why we highly recommend that you make your own alkaline water.

If you have more funds to support your alkaline water needs, then, by all means, you can get your own alkalized water. We recommend Essentia, which is 9.5 on the pH level, this is the bottled water you get, which is alkalized and all ready for you. Make sure that you use this water if you are looking to get more alkalized water in your body, however, if your goal is to make your own alkaline water and there are some ways to go about it. The way most people do it, is that use normal tap water they boil it making sure that they get rid of any pollution in the water. Let the water cool down, and then they will add minerals which they can easily be found online that will make the water even more alkaline.

Once they have done that, you will separately put it in a bottle and finally serve it when chilled. Utilizing this method will ensure they get rid of any pollutions in the water, and you will get a better pH level in the water as well. Your pH level should be around 9.2 to 9.5 if you use this method properly, giving you great alkalize water. However, if you live outside North American and European countries. Then there's a high chance that the water that you are getting from the tap is not drinkable, which is why you might have to spend a little bit more money on the alkaline water. Or you can buy machines which are known as water ionizer which will create alkaline water, and this method is called ionization. This could be an excellent idea for people who are living outside of North America and European countries to get the cheapest water source of the alkaline water.

With that being said, this should help you really understand how the alkaline water truly works and how you can use it for your own benefit. Let's talk about alkaline fruits and how can help you when it comes to bettering your health. As you know, there are many alkaline fruits, as you can refer to the chapter in the book where the talk about the whole section of which fruits are alkaline and which aren't. You will get a better idea on which fruits will help your body get alkaline even further, just like the water the alkaline fruits can genuinely help you with all the same benefits which the alkaline water can. In fact, once you combine the alkaline water alongside the alkaline fruits, you will see even better benefits when it comes to getting your body more alkaline and to see better health benefits overall. One of the great things about the alkaline fruits is that it always helps you with the bone density. It is essential that you take care of your bone density as it can cause a lot of issues if you don't, truth be told since you won't be eating a lot of dairies when following the alkaline diet. Getting a certain amount of calcium from your diet will drop down substantially.

Which is why it is highly recommended that you take bone support. You can take supplements, or it can come from the alkaline fruits that you are going to be eating. Many of the alkaline fruits include blueberries, watermelons, kiwi, etc. These fruits are known to help with bone density, which is why it is imperative that you eat these fruits when you're on the alkaline diet to see a better health benefit overall. Remember, the alkaline diet only works in a certain way; you need to have all aspects of this diet in check for it to work. You have to make sure that your diet is perfect, you have to make sure that you are on the alkaline side in the beginning by using the alkaline strips and finally you need to make sure that you are eating fruit to ensure that you are getting alkalized very quickly. With that being said, the take-home message from this chapter is that it doesn't matter if you drink alkaline water or you eat the alkaline fruit, everything needs to be in proper conjunction when it comes to seeing better results overall. With that being said, let us give you an example meal plan which will help you to get a better idea of how you should be eating

7 Day Eating Plan

Example meal plan

Monday

Breakfast - Wild rice cream of rice, almond milk, and berries

Snack - Green tea

Lunch - Salad with balsamic vinegar

Snack - Wild grain pita bread with hummus

Dinner - Plant-based meat substitute (found at a grocery store), cherry tomatoes and arugula.

Tuesday

Breakfast - Whole wheat pancakes or pancakes made from oats powders, served with berries and raw honey

Snack - Nuts and berries

Lunch - Sprouted beans and Greek salad

Snack - Almond butter, on wild grain bread

Dinner - Wild rice with beans boiled veggies (broccoli, asparagus, and spinach)

Wednesday

Breakfast - Egg substitute (in recipes chapter) with toast (whole wheat)

Snack - Smoothie with fruits and veggies

Lunch - Salad with beans and vegetables

Snack - Vegan protein

Dinner - Tofu Squeers (with your favorite herbs or spices) with wild rice and veggies

Thursday

Breakfast - Fresh veggie/fruit smoothie

Snack - Handful of trail mix

Lunch - Sprouted beans with boiled veggies and balsamic vinegar

Snack - Fruits

Dinner - Lentils and red onion with a dressing of extra-virgin olive oil with your favorite seasoning

Friday

Breakfast - Low sugar cereal almond milk and berries

Snack - Green tea

Lunch - Salad with balsamic vinegar

Snack - Pita bread with hummus

Dinner - Whole wheat bread with eggs substitute (in the recipes section) cherry tomatoes and arugula

Saturday

Breakfast - Wild rice cream of rice, with almond milk

Snack - Healthy smoothie

Lunch - Vegan protein shake with fruits

Snack - Almonds hand full

Dinner - Alkaline beans wild rice and a side of veggies and extra virgin olive oil.

Sunday

Breakfast - Whole wheat pancakes or pancakes made from oats powders, served with berries and raw honey

Snack - Vegan protein with fruits

Lunch - Vegan meat substitute, Greek salad

Snack - Almond butter, on whole wheat bread

Dinner - Sprouted with boiled veggies (broccoli, asparagus, and spinach)

Even though this chapter was on the longer side, we got a ton of things covered. Thank you so much for sticking thru this chapter and we will see you on the next one.

Chapter 6: Who and Why Should Follow Alkaline Diet

In this chapter, we are going to talk about who should be following the alkaline diet, and how it can benefit them depending on their goal. Evidently enough, many people have been starting to follow the alkaline diet for numerous reasons. More specifically, people follow the alkaline diet because they want to get rid of diseases, or not to attract them. This is one of the main things alkaline diet is known for, is to prevent diseases like cancer and many other harmful ones. Nonetheless, there are many other reasons why you should be following the alkaline diet to see optimal results and benefits. Which is what we're going to talk about in this chapter, we will talk about who should be following the alkaline diet and why should they be following it.

More specifically help you understand if the diet is right for you and your needs, as many people follow this diet for the wrong reasons. This is one thing we want to clear out before we move on, understand why you're following the alkaline diet and how it can help you. If you understand this concept and you will be a much better position in terms of getting the results that you're looking for with this diet. There are many benefits that you can see when the following alkaline diet, nonetheless there are many people following the alkaline diet for the wrong reasons. If you are someone looking to put on a lot of muscle, or to become a bodybuilder, for instance, then this diet will not be there right answer for you. Even though you can most definitely put on muscle following the alkaline diet, this diet will still not be ideal for those who are looking to compete professionally in bodybuilding or to put on an insane amount of muscle. Since this diet is vegan, you will have a hard time getting enough protein in, and on top of that, you should not be getting a lot of protein when you are following the alkaline diet anyways since you need to be on the alkaline side.

As explained to you, having a lot of protein in your diet can cause you to be more on the acidic side and therefore cause acidic imbalance. Also, if your goal is solely to look better or to look a certain way than the alkaline diet is not the right answer for you. You have to keep in mind that the alkaline diet can most definitely help you to lose weight and to look better. However, this isn't the main goal of this diet; the main goal of this diet is to help you to reduce the risk of diseases and to help you live healthier overall. One of the major things the alkaline diet helps you with is improving your kidney health; when you raise your pH level in your body, more specifically in your blood, you will improve your kidney health. In today's day and age, our kidney has not been taken care of properly, and more people are seeing chronic kidney diseases.

Therefore, the alkaline diet can help you too see better results and to keep your kidneys healthy overall. If you have any kidney issues, then the alkaline diet can most definitely help you to reduce that and to help you have a healthy kidney overall. When you're following the alkaline diet, your protein intake is going to be a lot lower as compared to normal Americans, which is why your kidney gets a major break from digesting all these proteins and therefore gives you a better healthy kidney. Another great benefit of the alkaline diet would be the fact that it helps you to get rid of cancer. However, this hasn't been proven, yet there have been many people claiming that it does. As we told you in the previous chapters that cancerous cells love the acidic environment, therefore if you put your body into an alkaline environment, the cells will not be able to live there and therefore die eventually. Which is one of the reasons why many people follow the alkaline diet tend to get rid of cancerous cells, if you're someone who's facing cancer or you are looking to get rid of cancerous diseases then, by all means, follow the alkaline diet. However, if you are going through chemotherapy, then make sure that you consult with your doctor before you start any diet, we cannot stress this enough.

Everybody's situation is a lot different when it comes to following a certain eating plan or following a certain diet. Another reason why the alkaline diet can help you to get rid of cancerous diseases is because of the fact that you will be eating a lot more fruits and vegetables, as you know eating a lot of fruits and vegetables has tremendous health benefits to our body. Since eating fruits and vegetables gives us the antioxidants that we need, we will be in a much better position of getting rid of cancerous cells and diseases. This one of the major benefits of the alkaline diet is to allow you to get all the micronutrients and antioxidants what you need, and quite frankly you're not getting it with your daily eating habits. Another great benefit of following the alkaline diet would be that it helps you to get rid of any heart diseases.

Many people who are facing heart diseases, or are looking towards preventing heart diseases than the alkaline diet can most definitely help you with that. There have been many studies showing that the alkaline diet had tremendous amounts of people to get rid of the heart diseases, more specifically lower their blood pressure. When you are eating foods, which are high in antioxidants, you will be lowering your blood pressure regardless, which is why the alkaline diet works so great and regards to reducing the risk of heart diseases, and to give you a better heart. One of the main things that the alkaline diet does is that it raises your growth hormone. When your growth hormone is raised, every bodily function gets better, which is why the alkaline diet works so great and giving a healthier body.

If your goal is to have a healthier better functioning body than the alkaline diet can most definitely help you to achieve that goal, just keep in mind that if you're a professional athlete, and you play a certain sport which needs you to put on a lot of muscle than the alkaline will not be the right answer for you. However, if you're happy with the muscular structure that you have for your sport or any athletic endeavors that you're doing, the alkaline diet can most definitely help you enhance your athletic performance. Many people don't know this, but, the alkaline diet has shown to improve peak performance in athletes. Studies have shown that when athletes follow the alkaline diet, their peak performance goes up, and they can sustain it for a longer period of time. Another great benefit of following the alkaline diet is that it lowers your inflammation levels, if you are someone who's facing a lot of information issues, then chances are that you're very acidic.

This is where the alkaline diet comes in, if you want to get rid of anybody pain which you're facing then the alkaline diet would be a great idea for you to follow. Many people who follow the alkaline diet reduce their back pain; their knee pain has gone away simply by following the alkaline diet. If you are someone who's facing these issues, then really consider the alkaline diet as it can truly work for you. The alkaline diet has also shown to reduce the risk of osteoporosis since alkaline diet helps you to strengthen up your bones, the risk of osteoporosis goes down. Another great benefit of following the alkaline diet is that it helps you to rejuvenate your cells, many people don't know this, but the alkaline diet helps you with autophagy which is the same process that many people see when following the intermittent fasting.

This process works so well that it essentially gets rid of your bad cells and rejuvenate it with new ones, if you are someone looking to detox your body the right way then you most definitely need to take care of your body by getting rid of any old cells. The only two diet's which help with autophagy is intermittent fasting and the alkaline diet. Now that you've gotten the idea on who should follow the alkaline diet, let's talk about the people who shouldn't follow the alkaline diet or follow it for the wrong reasons. If you are someone who's facing diseases, and you're solely banking on the alkaline diet helps you to get rid of it, then you are not the right person for this diet. Even though many people claim that this diet helps them to get rid of cancer, and many other diseases, that does not mean that you will get rid of your diseases by following the alkaline diet. Time and time again, many people think the alkaline diet is going to save them from everything which is simply not the case.

You have to consider the alkaline diet is a tool, the alkaline diet or work tremendously when it comes to helping you supplement your habits and other medications that you're taking to get rid of your diseases. However, this will not be the sole purpose of this diet. If you want to get rid of your diseases, always consult with the doctor position before you try anything as your case might be different than the others. If you're someone looking to follow this diet simply to lose weight, the chances are you will not see great benefits out of it. Since this diet essentially forces you to lose body fat, that does not mean it would be ideal for you and your needs. Keep in mind that people who are looking to lose weight can lose weight regardless of the diet that they're following, as long as they're in a caloric deficit, which is why this diet is not ideal for people who are looking to lose weight as it could be very restricting for them and quite frankly and not the right option. If you're someone who's never followed a diet before, the chances are this diet will not be the right answer for you. This diet can be difficult to follow; you will not be able to keep up with it if your primary goal is to lose weight.

Eventually, you'll find something else which will help you to lose weight and not see the benefits at all from the alkaline diet, which brings me to another point, if you're a beginner and you're looking to follow the alkaline diet, then do not follow it as you will not be able to keep up with it. If you have never restricted your diet ever in your life, the alkaline diet will be hard for you to continue. Make sure that you have some experience with restricting some foods before you start following the alkaline diet. Also, if you're someone looking to become a bodybuilder or a powerlifter, then chances of you seeing benefits from the alkaline diet would be slim to none, keep in mind that the alkaline diet is essentially made for people who are looking to better their health internally and externally. It is not meant to take things to the extreme like many bodybuilders and powerlifters are known to do, with that in mind you will have to disregard the alkaline diet if you're a bodybuilder or a powerlifter looking to see the benefits out of it. Hopefully, that makes sense to most people who are looking towards following this diet, as we talked about previously the people that will benefit the most from this diet are people who are looking towards reducing the risk of diseases or to live a healthier lifestyle internally and externally allowing them to live a longer life. With that being said, you should now have a clear idea on who should be following the alkaline diet based on their goals.

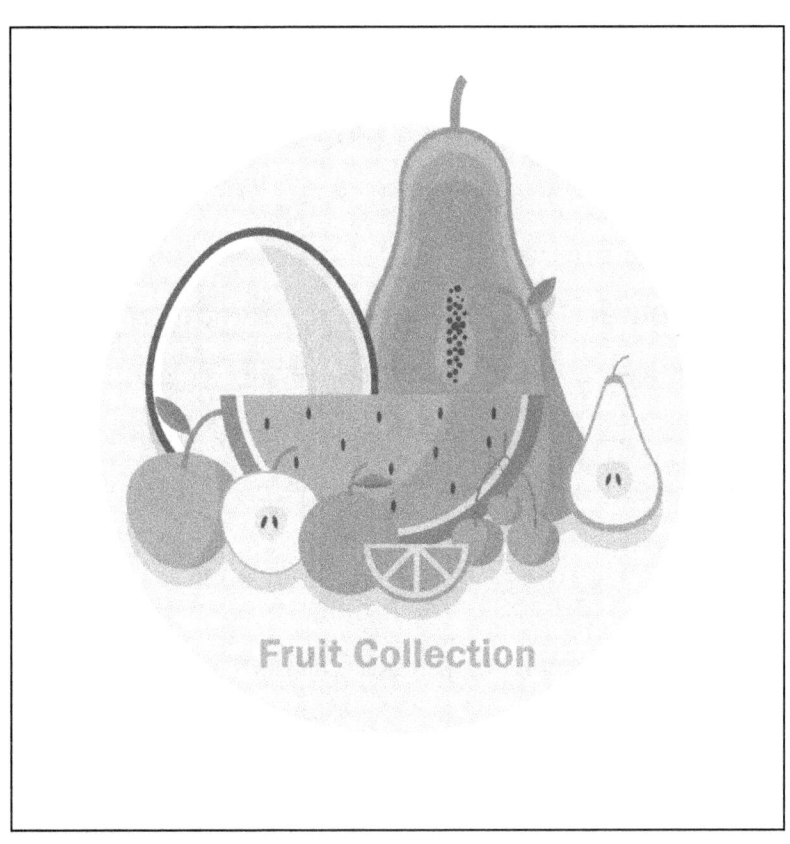

Chapter 7: How to Live the Lifestyle

We will talk about what you should be doing, to make sure that you are not failing in your endeavors to start this diet to live a healthier life overall. This chapter will show you what you could be doing to make this diet your lifestyle and to not only help you to start the Alkaline diet and stay on track but also to live with this eating plan for the rest of your life. These daily patterns will help you to not fail on your diet, and we understand that you might fail a couple of times in any diet, and it is understandable to do so. Nonetheless, this chapter will show you how to make sure you are consistent and not failing. These habits have been followed by many successful people, to get optimal results in all of their aspects of life, whether it is fitness related or anything else. Make sure you start implementing all of these habits after you are done reading this book as it will help you to make this diet your lifestyle. The reason why this chapter might sound philosophical is that the only way you will see success with this diet is if you do it consistently. For you to do that, you need to change your current lifestyle by being more productive and disciplined. You have to remember, healthy eating is more than just a meal; it's a lifestyle.

Plan Your Day Ahead

Planning your day ahead of time is crucial, not only does planning out your day help you be more prepared for your day moving forward, but it will also help you to become more aware of the things you shouldn't be doing, hence wasting your time.

Moreover, planning your day will truly help you with making the most out of your time, that being said, we will talk about two things 1. Benefits of planning out your day 2. How to go about planning out your day. So without further ado, let us dive into the benefits of planning out your day.

It Will Help You Prioritize

Yes, planning out your day will help you prioritize a lot of things in your day to day life. You can allow time limits to the things you want to work on the most to least, for example, if you're going to write your book and you are super serious about it. Then you need a specific time limit every day in which you work on a task wholeheartedly without any worries of other things until the time is up. Then you move on to the next job in line, so when you schedule out your whole day, and you give yourself time limits, then you can prioritize your entire day. The same thing goes for your diet, make sure you allocate time for prepping your meals for the next day, which will allow you to have meals ready for you when you need it hence making it easy for you to continue with your diet.

Summarize Your Normal Day

Now, before we start getting into planning out your whole day ahead, you need to realize that to plan your entire day, you need to know precisely what you are doing that day. Which means you need to write down every single thing you do on a typical day and write down the time you start and end, it needs to be detailed in terms of how long does it take for your transportation to get to work, etc.

Now after you have figured out your whole day, you can decide how to prioritize your day moving on could be cutting out a task that you don't require or shortening

114

your time for a job that doesn't need that much time. After you have your priorities for the day, you can add pleasurable tasks into your day like hanging out with your friends, etc.

Arrange Your Day

It is crucial that you arrange your day correctly, so the best way to organize your day is to make sure you get all your essential stuff done earlier in the day when your mind is fresh. After that's done, you can have some time for yourself to relax and do whatever it is that you want. But make sure you get all the things that need to be done before you can move on to free time for yourself. Another thing that will help you is to set time limits on each task, and once you start setting time limits, you will be more likely to get the job done.

Remove All the Fluff

So, what I mean by that is remove all the things that are holding you back from achieving your goals. Make sure you remove all of the things that are holding you back from getting the things that you need to be doing. If you have time for the fluff, do it if not, then work on your priorities first. In conclusion, planning out your day will help you tremendously! Make sure you plan out your day every day to ensure successful and accomplished days.

Cut Out Negative People

This task might be the hardest to do, but it is quite essential, see the people who you are around are the people who will create your personality. So if you are around negative people, you will develop adverse circumstances for yourself, so if you are around people who are not upbeat about life and find everything wrong and never see the good in anyone, you need to cut them out and be around people who are happy and ready for what life has to offer. Now I get it, some cynical people can be your family members, and you can't cut them out, the best thing to do is 1. Make them understand what they are doing wrong 2. Show them how they can change their life. And if they still want to remain the same, then keep your distance.

In conclusion, it is essential that you are in a grateful "vibe" as it will not only help you with your mental and physical health, but it will also help you attract better people and better circumstances. Don't forget to practice the three methods we discussed in this chapter for you to be in a grateful 'vibe" throughout the day and life! That being said I hope this chapter shed some light on the importance of being grateful and how it can make or break your life, and I hope you don't take this chapter lightly being grateful is the most critical thing you can do to turn your life around. So be thankful!

Now that we have covered the part of being grateful, and how it can help you with your day to day life and eating habits. Let us give you some concrete ideas on how to change the way you live your experience and to make it better.

Stop Multitasking

I think we are all guilty of this at a time, and if you are multitasking right now, I need you to stop. Now multitasking could be a lot of things, and it could be as small as cooking and texting at the same time, or it could be as big as working on two projects at the same time. Studies are showing how multitasking can reduce your quality of work, which something you don't want to do if your goal is to get the best result out of the thing that you are doing. That being said, there are a lot more reasons as to why you shouldn't be multitasking, so without further ado, lets dive into the primary reasons why multitasking can be harmful.

You're Not as Productive

Believe it or not, you tend to be a lot less productive when you are multitasking. When you go from one project to another or anything else for that matter, you don't put all your effort into your work. You are always worried about the project that you will be moving into next. So moving back and forth from one project to another will affect your productivity if you want to get the most out of your work you need to be focused on one thing at a time and make sure you get it done to the best of your abilities. Plus, you are more likely to make mistakes, which will not help you work at the best of your ability.

You Become Slower at Your Work

When you are multitasking, chances are you will end up being slower at completing your projects. You would be in a better position if you were to focus on one project at a time instead of going back and forth, which of course helps you complete them faster. So the thing that enables you to be faster at your projects when you're not multitasking is the mindset, we often don't realize how much mindset comes into play. When you are going back and forth from one project to another, you are in a different mental state going into another project which takes time to build and break. So by the time you have managed to get into the mindset of project A you are already moving into project B, it is always best that you devote your time and energy one project at a time if you want it to doe did an at a faster pace.

Set Yourself a Goal (Time, Quality, Etc.)

All in all, multitasking will do you no good. It will only make you slower at your work and make you less productive. Making sure you stop multitasking is essential, as it will only help you live a better life. One thing to remember from this chapter is to put all your energy at one thing at a time, and this will yield you a lot better projects or anything that you are working towards to be great. If you want to be more successful and live a better life, you need to make sure your projects are quality as I can't stress this point enough. You are probably reading this book because you want to get better at living your life or achieve goals which you haven't yet. One of the reasons why you are not living the life that you want or haven't reached your goal could be a lot of things but, one of the items could be the quality of your work which could be taking a hit because of your multitasking. So review yourself, and find out why you haven't achieved your goal and why you are not living the life that you want.

Then if you happen to stumble upon multitasking being the limiting factor or the quality of your work, I want you to stop multitasking and start working on one project at a time while giving it your full attention. What you will notice is that your work will have a higher quality and will be completed in a quicker amount of time following the steps listed above, which will change your life and help you achieve your life goals in a better more efficient way.

Now that we have talked about some action items in regards to making this diet more of a lifestyle by changing the way you set up your day. Let us talk about some of the lifestyle changes you need to make, in regards to making this alkaline diet more potent.

Get More Sleep

It is essential that you start getting your 8 hours of sleep. Many people don't know this but, even if your diet is perfect but you still aren't getting the sleep chances are you are not going to see the changes. Getting your 8 hours of sleep helps you a lot. When you get the right amount of deep sleep, you will see results such as better recovery and better mental health. It is essential that you get your full 8 hours of sleep if you don't, then this diet won't do its best for you in terms of results. Not only that, if you don't get enough sleep, the chances of you staying alkaline will drop down tremendously. You will be a lot more acidic the days you don't get your full sleep. Keep that in mind moving on, and as always make sure to get your total 8 hours of sleep.

Physical Activity

It is very crucial for you to take part in physical activities, for a straightforward reason it will help you to assist your alkaline diet. The same thing as getting proper sleep, the role of you being physically active will give you a great balance of you being alkaline throughout the day. Many people don't know this, but being physically active can help you to stay more alkaline. There have been many studies backing these claims up, that being said, let's talk about some of the benefits which might come along with you following the alkaline diet and working out.

Regular Exercising Changes Your Brain
No, regular exercises do not change the way your brain is shaped by any means if that's what you're thinking. But what it will help with, is better memory and better-thinking skills. If you were to do your research, you will find that out for yourself, how big of a role regular exercising plays when it comes to brain functions. Make sure you start implementing this physical activity, it will only help you get better at your alkaline diet and for you to see better results out of it.

By now you can see the benefits of exercising with you following the alkaline diet, not only does regular exercising help you stay healthy physically, but it also enables you to optimize your mind and helps you with better brain function which will allow you to work for an extended period at any given task.

Improves Your Mood

This is one of the most significant differences you will notice once you start working on your health is that your mood will stay elevated through the day! Which is a great thing to have as you will be able to get more things done and be more successful. See when you work out you release a chemical called dopamine, which is a feel-good hormone and of course working out will help you become less stressed.

Improves Physical Health

Yes, this is one of the most salient points to bring up but let's discuss it anyway. Once you start to implement healthy habits to your day you will become more physically healthy, which will not only give you more energy through the day it will also help you keep up with things like your daily chores and not get tired so quickly. You will see a difference in the quality of your life and your work ethic once you start to implement daily health habits and become more physically healthy.

Helps Boost Your Immune System

This ties into improved physical health, but working out will boost your immune system and lower your risk of diseases like diabetes, hypertension, etc. Once you have a boost in your immune system, you will be less likely to get even the common flu. I know of someone who hasn't gotten flu in fifteen years simply because he started to live a healthy life, now I am not saying that you will see the same results but staying healthy will definitely help you with boosting your immune system which will help you not get sick so often and enjoy some quality time with your family and get more stuff done.

Now that we have discussed how staying in shape can help you live a better life; we will now move on to the ways you can help yourself live a healthier life.

Start Easy

Now, if you have never worked out in your life, you need to realize that you won't be going hard at the gym as Arnold Schwarzenegger did in his hay days. So don't push yourself too much in the gym because you are not ready for it, and you might lose motivation. So if you are starting off getting in shape perhaps light jogs, some resistance training couple times a week to get the blood moving. But make sure you get up to the point where you are working out at least three hours a week to see some health benefits. Start once a week then twice, and so on.

After reading this chapter, many might be thinking that this is more of a self-help book than it is a diet book. The Truth is that we want you to understand how to live a better life by changing the habits that you are currently following. Following a diet and making it a lifestyle is a lot more work than you think it is. For you to make it easy, you need to understand that you need to change your habits in order to be successful at this diet, which means you need to change the way you move the way you think and the way you perform. This chapter gives you a clear idea on how to start living a better life by changing up your habits, once you do change your practices you will notice that following the Alkaline diet as a whole will be very easy for you.

The reason why it will be straightforward for you is that you will change the way you move and the change the way you live your life in general. Changing the way you live your life will not only help you get better results, but it will also help you to follow this diet as a lifestyle, many people confuse diet as not being a part of a lifestyle, and it is something that they're supporting to better their health. But the Truth is that when they're following a diet, they don't realize that it needs to be a lifestyle for it to be a health benefit, if you want to be healthier then you need to make sure that you're taking care of your health 24/7 365 days a year.

Which means you need to make this a lifestyle, and for you to make this a lifestyle, we need to understand some self-help techniques to keep it sustained for a more extended period. Which is why this chapter is more self-help oriented, we wanted to make sure that this book is different than any other books that you've read when it comes to following the Alkaline diet. The way we're going to be delivering it is by showing you how to change your lifestyle for the better instead of the worst. We're not just going to give you foods to eat and how to follow the Alkaline diet, but in fact, we're going to change the way you eat overall and to make it a better experience for you once you start getting into this diet. With that being said, I hope this chapter was helpful to you, and we will see you in the next chapter.

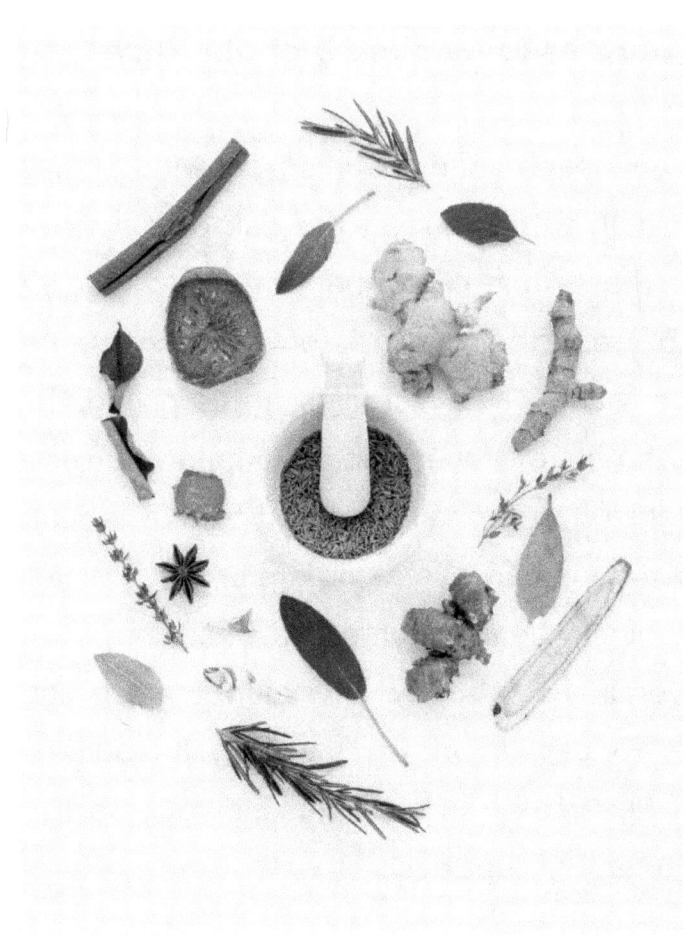

Chapter 8: Alkaline Diet and Diseases

There have been many studies showing that Alkaline diet can help with reducing the risk of cancer, which is why this diet is one of the best things to follow when it comes to reducing the risk of any disease that you might be facing. Many studies are showing that most people who have cancer and start following the alkaline diet fought off cancer and started to live a healthy life. Which is why we always recommend that you follow the alkaline diet when it comes to reducing the risk of cancer, or if you already have cancer, you can follow this diet to get rid of it. However, if you are facing cancer, then make sure to consult your doctor before you make any abrupt decisions.

The reason why the Alkaline diet works so well when it comes to reducing the risk of cancer is it because it lowers your acidic level. When you have lower acidic levels, there's a less chance of your body attracting more foul bacteria in your body which will cause cancer. This environment will discourage any cancer surviving growth, which is why many people recommend you follow an alkaline diet. Some people might say the alkaline diet is not the right answer when it comes to reducing the risk of cancer, in fact, most people said as long as you eat healthy foods then you will reduce the risk of cancer. However, many studies are showing that your lung and your other organs might be higher in the acidic level, which is why you're attracting more cancer in your body. The main thing you need to understand when it comes to reducing the risk of cancer is that cancer likes to thrive on acidic levels.

If your body is very acidic, you will be in a higher risk of attracting cancer regardless, which is why the alkaline diet works so well at reducing the risk of cancer. Moreover, people have also shown to reduce the risk of inflammation, which makes it a great idea to follow the alkaline diet when it comes to reducing the risk of cancer. As you might or might not know, one of the main reasons why we attract cancer is the inflammation in our body. Many people get cancer because they are inflamed, and it's causing issues overall increasing the risk of cancer. Once people start losing the inflammation in the body, the risk of cancer lowers even further making it a great idea to start following the alkaline diet as the alkaline diet reduces the risk of cancer and inflammation in your body. Also, as you know, the alkaline diet has shown to rejuvenate our body. Once you start to break down your old cells and come out with new ones, your body will have more fighting power towards the cancerous cells.

It is making the Alkaline diet one of the best diets to follow when it comes to reducing the risk of cancer. If your goal is to live a healthier life, then one of the main things you need to understand is your body recycling and detoxifying it very quickly. Which is where the alkaline diet comes on, any time you detoxify your body will be in much better shape to get rid of any diseases more specifically cancer. Anyhow, many people go on fasts and other things to detoxify the body. Which can also come in handy when it comes to reducing the risk of cancer, but the way this diet works is so perfectly that does not only detoxify your body but also makes it an alkaline environment where bacteria which cause cancer cannot survive. Also, when you are eating these high Alkaline foods, you're not only making it better for yourself to reduce the risk of cancer. You are also making your body more bacteria-friendly, as you will be adding more good bacteria in your body, helping you fight off the harmful bacteria in your body. As you might know, we have two types of bacteria in our body, and we have the good ones and the bad ones. We ideally want good bacteria in your body, to fight off any disease that we might notice. Which means you need to make sure that you have good bacteria in your diet. As you know, the alkaline diet provides you with good bacteria and lots of it. However, it would be best if you made sure that when you have these good bacteria is in your body that you are drinking enough water to digest it and to keep your gut healthy.

Which is why it is essential that you drink more alkaline water, which we will talk about that later in this book. However, for now, you need to understand the importance of good bacteria in your body and reducing cancer, overall if your goals to minimize cancer and alkaline diet will provide you with that. However, if your goal is to reap all the benefits from the alkaline diet, then you need to make sure that a couple of things are in check before you do so. You need to make sure they get an ample amount of protein, fats, and carbs in your diet. As your diet will be very restricted when it comes to the food you are going to be eating, you need to make sure that you are eating the right macronutrients for your body. Which means, we need to make sure that you are eating foods which will give you a balanced macronutrient breakdown.

You will be eating no meat, which means you'll have to make up your protein needs are met through plant-based meals and plant-based products. We will give you some fantastic recipes to make good food. However, your goal is to understand that you are hitting the right number of calories for your required body fat on your goals. If you're not eating an ample amount of food, then your body will not have enough energy to fight off these diseases or problems. Which is why you need to understand how many calories you need and eat accordingly based on that. Some people are claiming that you need to be eating enough food regardless of how much or what type of food intake you are following, which means that it is more recommended that you eat enough food to get the optimal results. If you're going through chemotherapy, then you need to be making sure they are eating enough food regardless of what diet you are following. If you want to make sure that your chemotherapy goes successful, then it is crucial that you maintain your weight when you are going through this procedure.

There are some claims made that the alkaline diet will make it more successful for you when it comes to achieving chemotherapy success. However, many people are claiming this is entirely bogus. No claims are backing up that Alkaline diet helps with chemotherapy. However, many claims are suggesting that the alkaline diet will help you with reducing the risk of cancer and are getting rid of cancer entirely if you are following the diet. If you talk to your doctor, he or she will tell you that the alkaline diet is one of the best diets to follow when it comes to reducing the risk of cancer. However, this is not the popular answer for most people.

As many people have been brainwashed with media saying that alkaline diet is not the best way to go about, if the professionals are saying that the alkaline diet is a great idea, there's some truth behind that. To clarify, there have not been many studies claiming that the alkaline diet will ultimately help you get rid of cancer. Nonetheless, there have been many real-life situations where this diet has helped.

If you want to make sure that you are getting the best results possible, then make sure that you combine it with a good smoothie routine which will allow you to detoxify your body. It doesn't matter what diet you follow. If you aren't following the alkaline diet or your body is alkaline, then there's a high chance that you will not reduce the risk of cancer. Which means you will be in a much better position following the alkaline diet when it comes to reducing the risk of cancer, many professionals have claimed as such. One more thing to remember, if you're on acidic medications then you can counteract that with an alkaline diet. Make sure that the medicines that you're taking aren't going to disrupt your alkaline diet. We can't tell you which medicine will cause you to be acidic, the best way to understand which ones will is to ask your doctor.

To recap, the alkaline diet will help you keep your body at an alkaline level, which will allow no cancer or bacteria to start activating or to start forming. The alkaline diet will detoxify you and create new cells which will enable you to fight off cancer and make your immune system even stronger. Moreover, the alkaline diet will also help you with chemotherapy, as many people have said it will. Making this diet a no-brainer to follow. Just make sure that you are eating enough calories to maintain your body weight, especially if you are facing any cancerous diseases. I hope you understand how following the alkaline diet can help you with reducing the risk of cancer and many other diseases, to clarify there have been no studies showing that the alkaline diet will help you to get rid of cancer or any other sorts of diseases.

This has been a personal recommendation of many doctors, and an own review of many patients that the alkaline diet has helped them tremendously to reduce the risk of cancer or many other diseases, which does make sense when you look at the benefits of the alkaline diet. If you're facing any of these diseases, then always consult with your doctor before you start any of this diet. Moreover, as always, know what type of medications you are taking and how can counterbalance your alkaline diet. Finally, truly understand what the alkaline diet is if you have to read this book a couple of times if you are feeling lost.

If you were going to follow this diet blindly, then it would be like riding a bicycle without training wheels. You need to understand the diet before you start following it, and feel it out before you can commit to it. If you can commit to this diet, then you will be in a great position in terms of seeing the benefits. One of the only problems with this diet would be the precise requirements. Also, you cannot drink alcohol or take any particular types of medication when following the alkaline diet. Make sure they have everything checked before you proceed to follow this diet. Once you have managed to do that, then you will be in a perfect position to start following this diet and to see the benefits of it.

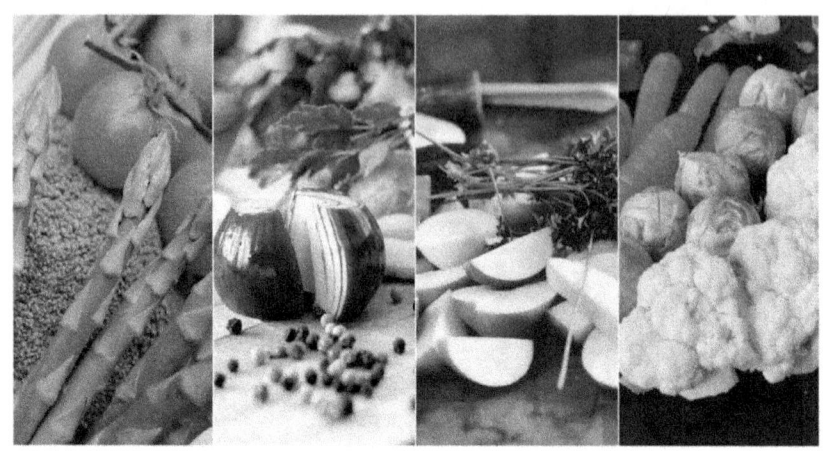

Chapter 9: Microbiome and Alkaline Diet

The Alkaline diet plays a huge role when it comes to your diet, many people don't know this, but the alkaline diet is known to be one of the easiest diets to follow. There's a reason behind that, especially with the foods that you're going to be eating when following the alkaline diet, digestion becomes very easy. Which is why you need to understand how the alkaline diet can really help you with digestion, that is what exactly we're going to be talking about in this chapter. More often than not, many people don't know this but as humans are not accustomed to consuming a lot of foods which we are eating as of right now. Which is why many people have digestion issues on leaky gut. One of the biggest issues many North Americans are facing with digestion, more specifically with the leaky gut.

Many people who don't know what leaky gut is, so let me explain that to you briefly. When you have small microscopic holes in your digestive system, which causes your gut to leak out acids and therefore cause you to it digest your food a lot less efficiently. 98% of the people in the world have a leaky gut; the good news is that you can fix it. One of the many ways to fix the leaky gut would be to pick out the right foods that you're going to be eating, and also to eat food, which is a lot less acidic. One of the many benefits people notice once they start following the alkaline diet is that the digestion gets a lot better, thanks to the alkalinity of the foods when following the alkaline diet.

Another thing to consider when fixing your digestion is that you need to have a certain number of good bacteria in your gut to help your food digest. Which is also going to come from the dense foods you're going to be eating when following the alkaline diet, overall having good health. This is very important not only for overall well-being but for you to have better digestion health overall.

With that being said, let's specifically talk about how the alkaline diet can help you with food digestion and leaky gut problems. Many people don't know this, but our body is not accustomed to eating meat, especially our gut. More often than not, many people do not have the enzymes to digest meat which is why many people are noticing gut issues especially in the North American countries were a lot of meat consumption is taking place. Us humans we are born herbivorous, which is why we don't have the enzymes to digest meat. It takes a special enzyme for us to digest meat, mostly carnivorous animals tend to have this enzyme in them. Having specific enzymes are essential when it comes to the food we are eating, which is we can't consume some foods, which is why we cannot consume meat since we don't have the enzymes to digest it.

Making the alkaline diet one of the top diets to follow when it comes to making the food we are to be eating, very accessible to us when it comes to digesting food. Not only that, since we are consuming a lot of foods that are going to be healthy and alkaline leaky gut issues are going to be gone. Let's talk about in a microbiome; it is essentially microorganisms present in your stomach which allow you to digest your food and to have healthier digestion. Now there are also unhealthy or toxic organisms in your body, which is also something the alkaline diet helps you to get rid of it.

Believe it or not, once you start drinking alkaline water, it will create a great place for good organisms to start living and to get rid of the toxic organisms. As we told you previously, bad toxins do not like alkaline situations, which is why the alkaline water will work so well when it comes to getting rid of it. There have been many scientific studies showing that the alkaline diet can help you tremendously to create a healthier environment for your gut, as you will digest food easily when following the alkaline diet your body will be a much better position to digest it. Many people have digestion issues because they don't understand their physiology, humans we are not meant to eat meat which is why we have a lot of gut issues since we're trying to digest a certain amount of food that we can't handle. We are not omnivores we are in fact herbivores, which is why you need to stop eating meat regardless if you follow the alkaline diet or not.

If you keep eating meat, then chances are you will become very toxic internally, and perhaps shorten your lifespan. Which is one of the reasons why you need to stop eating meat as because we're not built for it you are putting too much pressure on our body by eating it, when you have a vegan diet and conjunction with focusing on your alkalinity you will be in a much better position on keeping your leaky gut out of the system and to have a better digestion system overall. Not only that, since you'll be getting a lot of fiber when following the alkaline diet, your digestive system would really appreciate that in there or reward you with better digestive enzymes.

There have been such studies showing that eating a lot of fiber increases the good bacteria in your body and therefore helps you digest food a lot more efficiently, which is what you need to understand when you are following the alkaline diet. There are a lot of alkaline foods with a ton of fiber in them, so make sure you include them when you're following the alkaline diet. Overall this makes the alkaline diet one of the best diets out there in terms of bettering your results in and out of the body. The alkaline diet is more than just a diet it is a lifestyle, and we encourage you to appreciate it and use it for the right cause, which would be to help you to see better health benefits from it. With that being said, we come to a conclusion of this chapter. I hope this chapter was useful to you as it was for us to write it out. Make sure you read and understood this chapter as good as possible, so you know exactly why you are getting into the alkaline diet.

Conclusion

Thank you so much for downloading *Alkaline Diet for Beginners: The Best Guide to Understand PH; Learn How to Improve Your Weight Loss in A Healthy and Natural Way; Create A New Unlimited Energy Lifestyle To Reset and Cleanse Your Body*. As you can tell we learned a lot in this book, we learned many things such as how to follow the alkaline diet the right way, how to make this diet more attainable as a lifestyle for a very long period of time and finally how this diet can genuinely help you to change your life.

The alkaline diet is the answer for many questions you might be having in terms of health and wellness, but keep in mind that if the alkaline diet isn't for you, then it isn't for you. After reading this book, you should have a clear idea of whether this diet is the answer for you or not. If you are someone looking to get rid of diseases, or to lower the risk of diseases than the alkaline diet is for sure of the answer for you.

However, if you're following this diet just lose some weight, then make sure you get your priorities straight since this diet isn't the answer for you. Overall the alkaline diet will do nothing but good things for you, and as always consult with your doctor physician before you start any diet as we don't know how your body is feeling or what kind of reaction you might have when following this diet.

www.ingramcontent.com/pod-product-compliance
Lightning Source LLC
Chambersburg PA
CBHW060521290526
45791CB00001B/475